Diabetes Education
and
Prevention

Diabetes Education
and
Prevention
Instructional Module for Children

Adelia C. Bovell-Benjamin
and Rebecca Gyawu

TABLE OF CONTENTS

BACKGROUND

It has been predicted that there will be 552 million people, or one adult in 10 with diabetes in the world by 2030. In the Caribbean, type 2 diabetes is one of the leading health problems, contributing significantly to morbidity and mortality, and is more common in females than in males. The Republic of Trinidad and Tobago (Republic T&T) has one of the highest incidences of diabetes per capita in the western hemisphere. In the Republic T&T, diabetes is the second leading cause of death and the prevalence rate is approximately 12 to 13%. Diabetes is the leading cause of blindness and limb amputations in the Republic T&T.

It has been estimated by the Diabetes Association of Trinidad and Tobago (DATT) that in the Republic T&T, 175,000 persons have diabetes and 300 limbs are amputated annually because of diabetes. According to the Ministry of Health, Republic T&T, one adult in eight has diabetes, but not all of them know it. There are roughly 102,100 persons in the Republic T&T with pre-diabetes. This number is projected to increase to 130,500 by the year 2025. Research has indicated that in the absence of specific education programmes aimed at prevention or early detection, more than 50% of those persons with pre-diabetes will go on to full-blown diabetes.

There is compelling clinical proof that diabetes is largely preventable—80% of diabetes cases can be prevented, for example, by improving diets and increasing physical activity. Community-based diabetes education has the potential of reaching a relatively large number of people at a relatively low cost. At the same time, it may enhance diabetes awareness and prevention, while improving the behaviours and quality of life for those affected. The North American Caribbean Region (NAC) of the International Diabetes Federation (IDF) identified training and education as key challenges to diabetes prevention and management in the Caribbean Region. The current management of diabetes in primary care in the Republic T&T falls short of Caribbean guideline recommendations (Pereira et al., 2009).

Overall, many people in Republic T&T have undiagnosed diabetes, untreated diabetes, or are at high risk for developing diabetes, primarily because of lifestyle behaviours, genetics and lack of education about the condition. The link between diabetes and education is a key target for efforts to prevent, reduce the incidence and control diabetes-related complications in those individuals already diagnosed with the disease. If the burden of diabetes in the Republic T&T is to be effectively addressed, there is an urgent need to raise the level of knowledge regarding diabetes prevention and self-management among children and other community members in Tobago.

There has been growing concern about the recent increase in reported cases of Type 2 diabetes in children and adolescents. Several studies have demonstrated this increase worldwide. The diabetes prevention lessons that children learn when they are young will be carried into adulthood. Therefore, the overall purpose of the module is to educate children about diabetes with emphasis on type II diabetes, its prevention and control.

This module consists of eleven lessons, including a series of evaluation questions and a diabetes bingo. The lessons were created for 10 to 15 year-old children; however, teachers could always modify the contents to meet their specific groups of learners. The class time may also be adjusted accordingly. The module is suitable for use by diabetes educators, health educators, school teachers; community-based organisations (CBOs), non-governmental organisations (NGOs) health departments, nutrition units, faith-based organizations (FBOs) or any groups or persons involved in diabetes education and prevention efforts. The lesson content (for example, the food groups) could be modified to meet the needs of any community, region or country worldwide.

The Bovell Cancer Diabetes Foundation plays a unique and vital role in diabetes prevention, management and control via a structured, multi-faceted, diabetes education and prevention programme in Tobago, Republic of Trinidad and Tobago, West Indies. BCDF has a broad vision of enriching lives one person at a time, and its mission is enriching lives of people living with cancer and diabetes and those at risk, by providing financial resources, support, management and preventive education. To develop, implement and manage its programme, BCDF depends solely on volunteers, donations, fundraisers and proposal writing.

This publication was prepared by Adelia C. Bovell-Benjamin and Rebecca Gyawu. Information concerning the publication can be obtained from:

BACKGROUND

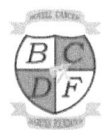 Bovell Cancer Diabetes Foundation (BCDF)
http://www.bovellcancerdiabetesfoundation.org
E-mail: adelia@bovellcancerdiabetesfoundation.org
Facebook: https://www.facebook.com/pages/Bovell-
CancerDiabetes-Foundation/1092530079221608

Bovell Cancer Diabetes Foundation
19 King Orange Avenue, South
Santa Rosa Heights
Arima
Republic of Trinidad and Tobago

BACKGROUND

CREDITS AND ACKNOWLEDGEMENTS

Adelia C. Bovell-Benjamin, PhD, CFS is a Professor of Food and Nutritional Sciences in the College of Agriculture, Environment and Nutrition Sciences (CAENS), Tuskegee University, Tuskegee, Alabama, U.S.A. and a Director on the Board of Directors of the Bovell Cancer Diabetes Foundation (BCDF). Professor Bovell-Benjamin has more than 30 years experience as a teacher/educator at all levels of the school system, from infants through university level; and has served in many capacities such as, Nutrition Educator and Community Nutritionist.

Rebecca Gyawu is a Master of Science Candidate in Food and Nutritional Sciences in the College of Agriculture, Environment and Nutrition Sciences (CAENS), Tuskegee University, Tuskegee, Alabama, U.S.A. Ms Gyawu holds a Bachelor of Education with emphasis on Food and Nutrition and has worked as a Teacher, Nutrition Educator and Counsellor in Ghana, West Africa.

The design on the front cover highlights drawings from the Bovell Cancer Diabetes Foundation 2011 Primary School Children Poster Competition and the layout was created by Professor Bovell-Benjamin. Several sources were utilised to complete this *module*, and the authors have been given credit at the end of the module.

LESSON ONE

<u>OVERVIEW OF NUTRITION—PART I</u>

Age level: 10-15 years   **Class time**: 45 minutes

<u>Teaching Objectives</u>

The objectives of this lesson are to:

◈ Differentiate between nutrients and nutrition
◈ Identify the major classes of nutrients
◈ Discuss the basic functions of foods
◈ Define a balanced diet
◈ State risk factors for chronic diseases including diabetes

<u>Learning Outcomes</u>

By the end of the lesson, students should be able to:

◈ Differentiate between nutrients and nutrition
◈ Identify six classes of nutrients in food
◈ Discuss at least three functions of food
◈ Define a balanced diet
◈ State at least three risk factors for chronic disease development

Materials Needed

Food samples: bread, potatoes, macaroni, oils, butter, margarine, milk, eggs, meat, fruits and vegetables

Introduction

Time allocated: 2 minutes

Teaching method: Riddle

Teaching activity:
- ◈ Teacher tells a riddle to introduce the topic for the lesson
- ◈ Teacher defines food

Summary

RIDDLE RIDDLE!!!

Class response: "SHALL BE"

Teacher continues with the riddle

I am the first thing you think about when you wake up in the morning, you need me to help you grow strong and healthy; without me, you become hungry and weak. WHO AM I?

ANSWER: *Food*

- ◈ Food is any nourishing substance, which when eaten provides energy, builds the body and protects the body from diseases to make us healthy.

Section A: Nutrients and Nutrition

Time allocated: 5 minutes

Teaching method: Lecture

Teaching activity:
- ◈ Define nutrients
- ◈ Define nutrition
- ◈ Differentiate between nutrients and nutrition

Summary

Nutrients are the components of food, which perform functions such as:

- Provide energy
- Sustain growth
- Protect against diseases

- Nutrition is the study of foods, how they are made up, and how each individual nutrient contributes to a person's overall health.

Differentiation

- Nutrients are the components of food and nutrition is the study of these components.

Section B: Classes of Nutrients

Time allocated: 6 minutes

Teaching method: Discussion

Teaching activity:

- Explain to students the classes of nutrients
- Using the food samples as examples, classify the nutrients

Materials needed:

Food samples (bread, potatoes, spaghetti, oils, butter margarine, milk, eggs, meat, fruits and vegetables).

Summary

Nutrients in food fall into these classes:

- Carbohydrates: example—bread, potatoes, macaroni, etc.
- Lipids (fats): example—oils, butter, margarine etc.

- ◈ Proteins: example—milk, egg, meat
- ◈ Vitamins: example—fruits and vegetables
- ◈ Minerals: example—fruits and vegetables
- ◈ Water
- ◈ Fibre

Section C: Reasons Why We Eat

Time allocated: 8 minutes

Teaching method: Class discussion

Teaching activities:

- ◈ Ask student questions
- ◈ Explain to them the role food plays in the body

Sample Questions:

1. *When you do not eat, how do you feel?*
2. *As soon as you eat, how do you feel?*
3. *So what does eating do for you?*

Summary

Food performs the following functions:

I. **Growth.** Food is essential for growth. Without food a living organism will stop growing. The living cells in our body multiply after getting nourishment from the food we eat. Insufficient or too much food does not help healthy growth.

II. **Repair.** Living organisms sometimes damage their parts by accident. Constant work also causes wear and tear of the body parts. If we get a wound or cut, it heals after some time. If we damage our skin due to some burn etc., it regains its shape in due course. The body needs food for all these functions.

III. **Energy.** We use energy to work, that is why we get tired. We then need food and rest to regain the lost energy. If we do not get food, we would become weak.

IV. **Protection from Disease**. We need to protect our body from diseases and keep it healthy. For this, we need vitamins and minerals from foods. Vitamins neither provide energy, nor do they repair or replace the worn-out parts; but they are essential in protecting our body against diseases.

So, we need food which can help us to grow, to repair our bodies, to give us energy, and protect us against diseases. We also need food in sufficient amounts—neither too much nor too little. That is to say, we should eat the right amount of food containing the right amount of nutrients.

Section D: A Balanced Diet

Time allocated: 3 minutes

Teacher method: Discussion

Teaching activity:

◈ Ask students sample question; then explain a balanced diet.

◈ *Sample question*: *What does it mean to eat a balanced diet?*

Answer/summary:

A balanced diet is one, which has all the nutrients such as protein, fat, and carbohydrates, required by a child in correct proportions for healthy growth.

Section E: Risk Factors of Chronic Disease

Time allocated: 6 minutes

Teaching method: Discussion

Teaching activity:

◆ Define chronic disease
◆ List some examples of chronic disease
◆ Discuss with students risk factors, which can lead to chronic disease development
◆ Encourage students to eat healthy

Summary

What do you understand when we say something is chronic?

Students respond

Define chronic disease

The term chronic disease commonly applies to conditions that can be treated, but not necessarily cured. Chronic disease means persistent or recurring diseases. Usually, chronic diseases are genetic or result from lifestyle factors. They are not contracted from another person, that is, they are non-communicable.

Examples of chronic disease

◆ Diabetes mellitus
◆ Arthritis
◆ Some types of cancer
◆ Heart disease
◆ Kidney disease etc.

Risk Factors for Chronic Disease

1. **Obesity and overweight**—Obesity is a term used when your range of body weight is greater than what is considered healthy for a given height. **Body**

mass index (BMI) is a measure used to determine childhood overweight and obesity. It is calculated using a child's weight and height. BMI does not measure body fat directly, but it is a reasonable indicator of body fatness for most children and teenagers. A child's weight status is determined using an age-and sex-specific percentile for BMI, rather than the BMI categories used for adults because children's body composition vary as they age, and vary between boys and girls. The **percentile** indicates the relative position of the child's BMI number among children of the same sex and age. Tables 1.1 and 1.2 and Figure 1.1 show cut-points for BMI, weight status and percentile range, and example of BMI samples for a 10-year old boy, respectively. Teacher explains tables and figure to students.

2. **Unhealthy diet:** a diet that fails to provide our body with the correct amounts and types of nutrient for maximum health. An example is a diet that contains too many calories, and not enough fruits and vegetables.

3. **Physical inactivity**: when one does not engage in any physical activity that requires the use of energy.

4. **Genetics**

5. **Smoking**

6. **Ethnicity**

Table 1.1. BMI Percentile Cut-Points (kg/m²)

Age (years)	Boys	Girls
5	20.1	21.5
6	21.6	23.0
7	23.6	24.6
8	25.6	26.4
9	27.6	28.2
10	29.3	29.9
11	30.7	31.5
12	31.8	33.1
13	32.6	34.6
14	33.2	36.0
15	33.6	37.5
16	33.9	39.1
17	34.4	40.8

Table 1.2. Weight Status and Percentile Range

Weight Status Category	Percentile Range
Underweight	Less than 5th percentile
Healthy weight	5th percentile to less than the 85th percentile
Overweight	85th percentile to less than the 95th percentile
Obese	Equal to or greater than the 95th percentile

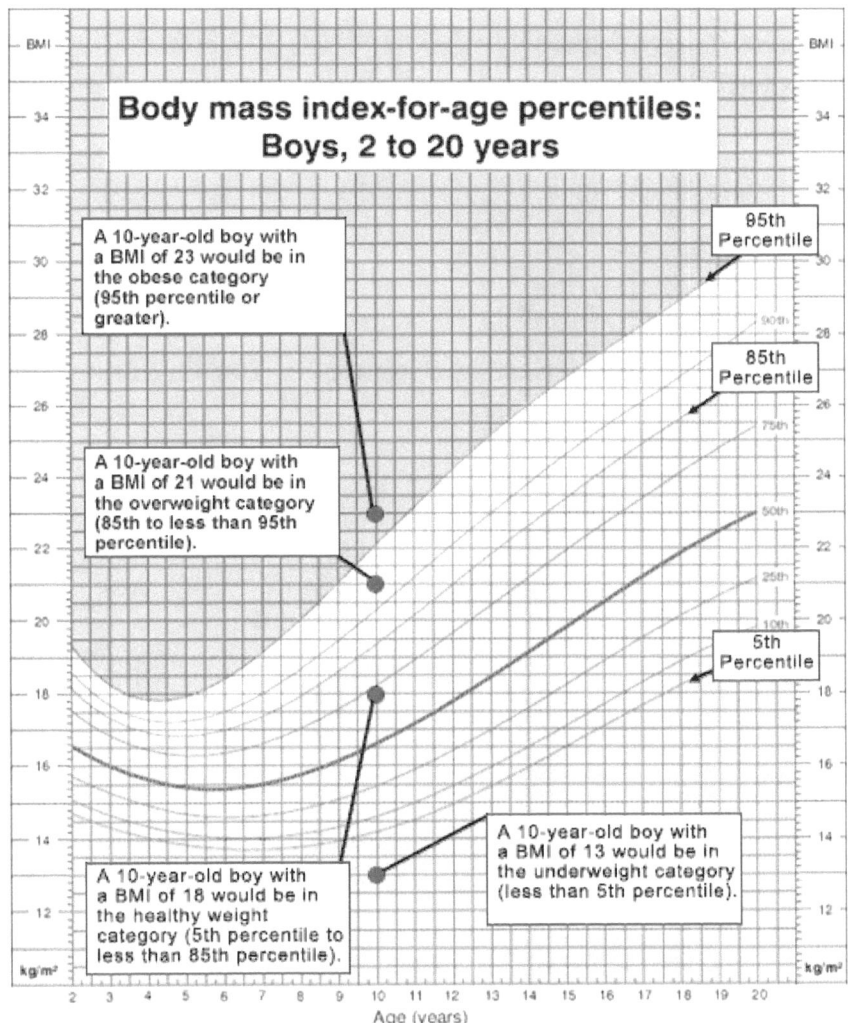

Figure 1.1. Interpretation of Sample BMI Numbers for a 10-year-old Boy

From: *http://www.cdc.gov/healthyweight/assessing/bmi/ childrens_bmi/about_childrens_bmi.html*

Evaluation: (see next page)

Time allocated: 10 minutes

Assignment: List and explain six functions of food in the body

Instruction: Assignment should be handed in by the next lesson

Closure:

Time allocated: 5 minutes

Activity: Teacher summarizes the lesson for the day and invites questions from students.

EVALUATION-OVERVIEW OF NUTRITION-PART I

Name: _____   Maximum points: 10

Instructions: Using this worksheet, answer all questions correctly

1. Nutrition is the study of foods and nutrients are the
   _____ in food.
   a. Components b. Compromises c. Confidences *1 point*

2. List the six classes of nutrients

   C _____   W _____
   P _____   V _____
   F _____   M _____   *4 points*

3. Foods perform all the following functions **EXCEPT**:
   a. Growth
   b. Repair
   c. Energize
   d. Operate
   e. Protect   *1 point*

Circle True or False for the sentence below:

4. A balanced diet contains all the nutrients in the right proportion and amount
   . . . True   . . . False   *1 point*

5. List six risk factors for chronic disease development
   3 points

   _____   _____
   _____   _____
   _____   _____

LESSON TWO

<u>OVERVIEW OF NUTRITION—PART II</u>
CARBOHYDRATES

Age level: 10-15 years   **Class time**: 45 minutes

<u>Teaching Objectives</u>

The objectives of this lesson are to:

1. Define carbohydrates
2. Explain the types of carbohydrates
3. Identify food sources of simple and complex carbohydrates

<u>Learning Outcomes</u>

By the end of the lesson students should be able to:

- Define carbohydrates
- Explain the different types of carbohydrates
- List at least three source of simple carbohydrates
- List at least three food sources of complex carbohydrates

Materials Needed:

Food samples or pictures of foods—sweets, cakes, syrup, bubble gum, soft drink, oatmeal, sweet potatoes, dried peas and beans, Kit Kat, wheat bread, white bread, ice cream and sweet biscuits, macaroni, corn

Introduction

Review previous lesson

Section A: *Definition of Carbohydrates*

Time allocated: 5 minutes

Teaching method: Lecture

Summary

Carbohydrates

Carbohydrates are macronutrients, which when eaten, are broken down into **glucose**. Glucose serves as the fuel, which gives our body energy and keeps us going. Glucose is the end product of carbohydrate breakdown. Carbohydrates contain **carbon, hydrogen and oxygen.** Carbon, hydrogen, and oxygen are tiny elemental particles that make up most living things. For this lesson we will think of them as building blocks that make up the nutrients found in food. In Figure 2.1, hydrogen is the tiny grey particles, the medium sized grey particles are oxygen, and the large blackish particles represent carbon. They link together in different ways like a rubrics cube to make many molecules. Teacher goes over the figure with students.

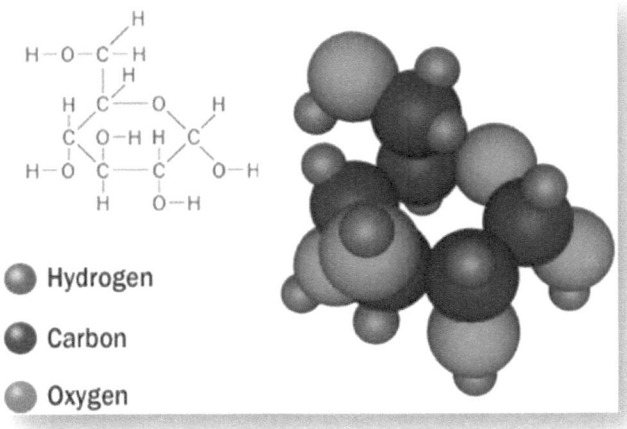

Figure 2.1. Molecular Construction of Glucose
Taken from: *Keckler, A. 2008. Nutrition: Carbohydrates. Available at http://www.annekeckler.com; accessed 7/4/2013*

SECTION B: *Types of Carbohydrates*

Time allocated: 10 minutes

Teaching method: Class discussion

Teaching activity:

◈ Explain to students the types of carbohydrates.

Summary

There are two types of carbohydrates

◈ Simple carbohydrates

◈ Complex carbohydrates

Simple carbohydrates are short chains of carbon, hydrogen and oxygen. They include sugars found naturally in foods, and they are quickly broken down into glucose and absorbed by the body. They can be found in foods such as ice cream, candies, soft drinks, etc.

Complex carbohydrates are long chains of carbon, hydrogen and oxygen. Your body takes longer to digest them than it takes to digest simple carbohydrates. As a result, digesting complex carbohydrates releases glucose into your bloodstream more slowly and evenly than digesting simple carbohydrates. They are not broken down quickly to produce energy. Complex carbohydrates include **starch** and **dietary fibre.**

◈ **Starch** must be broken down through digestion before the body can use it as glucose. Food sources of starch include: dried beans and peas, corn, bread, cereals, grains and sweet potatoes.

◈ **Dietary fibre** is found in vegetables, fruits and whole grain. They can be soluble or insoluble.

o   Soluble fibers are absorbed by the body and they can be found in foods such as oatmeal, most fruits, dried peas and beans etc.

o   Insoluble fibers are not digested and they can be found in foods such as wheat bran, whole wheat bread, brown rice etc.

We need to eat simple and complex carbohydrates to give our bodies energy. For every ten pieces of food we eat, about five and a half of them should contain carbohydrates for us to get the energy we need to grow and be active. Complex carbohydrates are more useful to us than simple carbohydrates because they allow our bodies to have more energy for a longer period of time.

If we do not have enough carbohydrates, our bodies can be affected. We get most of our body's energy from carbohydrates; if we do not get enough, our body systems can slow down, making us groggy and tired. **Glucose**, the very important simple sugar is needed to give the body energy; without it we can feel dizzy, weak, and may even go into a coma if we are diabetic. If we do not take carbohydrates in our diet, then our bodies will have to make glucose from other sources such as proteins and lipids (fats).

SECTION C: Food Sources of Simple and Complex Carbohydrates.

Time allocated: 10 minutes

Teaching method: Class discussion

Teaching activity

◈   Draw a table with two columns and seven rows on the board. Title the first Column *simple carbohydrates* and the second Column *complex carbohydrates* following the sample and list given below.

◆ Ask students to categorise the food samples from the list (more foods can be added to the list) into simple and complex carbohydrates as you write them on the chalk board.

Summary:

SIMPLE CARBOHYDRATES	COMPLEX CARBOHYDRATES

List: sweets, cakes, syrup, bubble gum, soft drink, oatmeal, sweet potatoes, dried peas and beans, Kit Kat, wheat bread, white bread, ice cream and sweet biscuits, macaroni, corn

Evaluation (see next page)

Time allocated: 10 minutes

Assignment: List ten sources/examples of:

a) simple carbohydrate

b) complex carbohydrate

Instructions: assignment should be ready before next lesson.

Closure

Time allocated: 10 minutes

Teaching activity: Teacher summarises the lesson and invites questions from students.

EVALUATION
OVERVIEW OF NUTRITION—PART II
CARBOHYDRATES

Name: _____   Maximum points: 10

Instructions: Answer all questions correctly

Circle True or False for the sentences below

1. Carbohydrate provides the
   body with energy.   . . . True   . . . False   *1 point*
2. Carbohydrates can be simple
   or complex.   . . . True   . . . False   *1 point*
3. Simple carbohydrates are quickly broken
   down to glucose.   . . . True   . . . False   *1 point*

Fill in the blanks

4. Complex carbohydrates include . . . . and . . . .   *1 point*
5. Dietary fiber can be classified as . . . . and . . . .   *1 point*
6. Using the food list and table below, classify the
   given foods as complex or simple carbohydrates.
   Food list: sweets, cakes, syrup, bubble gum, soft
   drink, oatmeal, sweet potatoes, dried peas and
   beans, Kit Kat, wheat bread, white bread, ice cream
   and sweet biscuits, macaroni, corn   *5 points*

SIMPLE CARBOHYDRATES	COMPLEX CARBOHYDRATES

LESSON THREE

<u>OVERVIEW OF NUTRITION—PART III</u>
<u>PROTEINS & LIPIDS (FATS)</u>

Age level: 10-15 years   **Class time**: 45 minutes

<u>Teaching Objectives</u>

The objectives of this lesson are to:

1. Define proteins
2. Explain the functions of proteins
3. Identify food sources of proteins
4. Define lipids
5. Explain the functions of lipids
6. Identify food sources of lipids

<u>Learning Outcomes</u>

By the end of the lesson students should be able to:

- Define proteins
- Explain the functions of proteins
- List at least five source of proteins
- Define lipids
- Explain the functions of lipids
- List at least five source of lipids

Relevant Previous Knowledge: Overview of Nutrition

Materials Needed: Pictures of food sources of proteins and lipids

Introduction

Review previous lesson "Overview of Nutrition"

Time allocated: 2 minutes

Section A: *Definition of Proteins*

Time allocated: 5 minutes

Teaching method: Lecture and learning activities

Summary

Proteins

Protein is one of the most important nutrients in food, because it is the chief constituent of the body cells, body tissues and body fluids. Proteins are very large molecules consisting of long chains of smaller units known as **amino acids**. Approximately 20 different amino acids are used in the production of proteins. Suppose that we let the letter **A** stand for one amino acid, the letter **B** for a second amino acid, the letter **C** for a third amino acid, and so on through the 20 amino acids. Therefore, **amino acids** are the building blocks from which proteins are made. Then one simple way to represent a section of a protein is as follows: -A-B-N-E-Y-W-C-K-S-R-I-A-J-B-D-S-K-H-S-E-H-C-A-I-E-F-M-Q-I-A-S—This representation actually shows only one small part of a protein molecule. Most proteins are very large molecules that contain hundreds or thousands of amino acids. Proteins are made up of:

➢ Carbon (C)

➢ Hydrogen (H)

➢ Oxygen (O)

➢ Nitrogen (N)

➢ and some proteins contain sulphur (S)

Proteins are special because they are the only nutrient, which contain **nitrogen**.

LESSON THREE

There are just over 20 naturally occurring amino acids. Most can be made by the body from other **substrates** (a biochemical word for reactants which react at the active site of an enzyme), though some cannot. Those that cannot be made by the body are called **essential amino acids,** because we <u>must</u> get them from the food we eat.

Section B: *Functions of Proteins*

Time allocated: 3 minutes

Teaching method: Lecture and activities

Summary

Proteins help us to grow and repair new tissues to keep our bodies healthy and growing strong. They also help our bodies to make **enzymes** and **antibodies**. Proteins also provide energy if sufficient carbohydrates and fats are not supplied by the diet.

LESSON THREE

What is an enzyme?

◆ Enzymes are substances used in the body to help us make changes in our bodies, like breaking down food.

What is an antibody?

◆ Antibodies are special enzymes that protect us from germs, which try to infect our bodies. We need them to stay healthy and well.

Section C: *Food Sources of Proteins*

◆ *Time allocated*: 10 minutes

Summary

Animal and Plant Proteins

Animal (Complete protein)

◆ Meat (beef, lamb, pork, goat meat etc.); poultry (chicken, duck, turkey etc.); fish; eggs; milk; cheese

Plant (Incomplete protein)

◆ Dried peas and beans (split peas, lentils; red beans, soya beans etc.); nuts (peanuts, red skins, cashew etc.). People who eat vegetarian diets will need to mix beans and grains to get all the essential amino acids that he or she needs to be healthy. This special type of combination of protein is called **complementary proteins**.

Teacher's activity to reinforce

◆ Hold up food pictures that are complete (animal) and incomplete (plant) proteins. Then put several foods together to simulate a complete protein.

    o   peas and macaroni

    o   peanut butter and whole wheat bread

    o   red beans and rice

LESSON THREE

- Extend plant proteins with small amounts of animal proteins:
    o chicken and rice
    o macaroni and cheese
- On chalkboard draw a ladder, with broken and missing rungs to represent incomplete proteins. Show how the ladder can be repaired.

When we have too little protein we can get **malnourished**. The muscles in our bodies get very small and weak as all the muscle protein is used up for other bodily functions—this is called **Marasmus**. A person with too little protein can have another disease where the stomach (belly) gets very rounded and swollen—this is called **Kwarshiorkor**. If we have too much protein in our diets, we can increase our risk for heart disease, cancer, osteoporosis and obesity.

Teacher activity to aid in understanding and reinforcement of the lesson

- Point out to the students that some foods contain complete (animal source foods) proteins and some foods contain incomplete (plant source foods) proteins. Guide the students to the understanding that whenever incomplete protein foods are eaten, they must be complemented (complementary proteins), or the amino acids will go unused and be excreted by the body. Pose the question, *"How can you correct for an incomplete protein food?"*

Section D: *Definition of Lipids (Fats)*
- *Time allocated*: 3 minutes
- *Teaching method*: Lecture

Summary
Lipids

Lipid is the scientific term used to depict fats and oils. The terms are interchangeable, but fats or oils are more commonly used in everyday language. At room temperature, oils are **liquids**, but fats are **solids**. A liquid is something that can flow and take on the shape of its container. Solids do not move freely unless a force like a push or pull is put on them, and they have a shape of their own at room temperature.

Section E. *Functions of Lipids (Fats)*

- ◈ *Time allocated*: 3 minutes
- ◈ *Teaching method*: Lecture

Summary

Lipids or fats perform a number of critical functions in the human body. These functions include:

1. Insulation
2. Repair of walls of arteries and veins
3. Energy storage
4. As a solvent for vitamins A, D, E, and K
5. They provide linoleic acids and calories (9 per gram).

Section F. *Food Sources of Lipids (Fats)*

- ◈ *Time allocated*: 3 minutes
- ◈ *Teaching method*: Lecture

Summary

Fats in our foods that come from plants are oils; that is, they are **liquid** at room temperatures. Examples are corn oil, vegetable oil, etc. Fats from animal source foods are generally **solid** at room temperature. The exception is vegetable shortenings, which are chemically modified plant oils that remain solid at room temperature. Solid lipids can be found in butter, lard, cheese etc. (Figure 3.2).

Fats should not be eaten in excess, and eating them in excess is easy to do in our culture, because they are such an integral part of our everyday food preparation and festivals such as Heritage Festival, Blue Food Festival etc.

Evaluation (see page 28)

Time allocated: 10 minutes

Assignment: List ten food sources/examples for:

  a) Proteins (animal and plant sources)
  b) Lipids (solid and liquid sources)

Instruction: assignment should be ready before next lesson

Closure

Time allocated: 6 minutes

Teaching activity: Teacher summarises lesson and invites questions from students.

MARGARINE
- 80% fats (vegetable), milk solids, water, salt, flavouring, coloring

SHORTENING
- All vegetable oil or combination of vegetable oils and animal fats
- Partially hydrogenated (a process which improves keeping quality and imparts shortening consistency)
- Small amounts of emulsifiers, preservatives, anti-foam agents

LARD
- 100% rendered pork fat, preservatives

BUTTER
- 80% butterfat, water, milk solids, salt

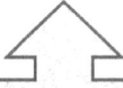

OIL
- All vegetable oils (small amount of preservatives, anti-foam agents, flavourings)

Figure 3.1. Some Common Fats and Oils

EVALUATION
OVERVIEW OF NUTRITION—PART III
PROTEINS AND LIPIDS

Name: _____   Maximum points: 20

Instructions: Answer all questions correctly

Circle True or False for the sentences below

1. There are animal and plant sources
   of protein.   . . . True   . . . False   *1 point*
2. Protein is essential to
   good health.   . . . True   . . . False   *1 point*
3. Protein always means
   red meat.   . . . True   . . . False   *1 point*
4. Fats in our foods that come from plants are liquid
   at room temperature.   . . . True   . . . False   *1 point*
5. Vegetable shortenings, which are
   plant oils remain solid at
   room temperature.   . . . True   . . . False   *1 point*
6. A liquid is something that can flow and take on the
   shape of its container.   . . . True   . . . False   *1 point*
7. List three reasons why protein is needed by the
   body.   *3 points*

   a. _____

   b. _____

   c. _____
8. Complete the chart by listing as many foods containing
   protein as you can. Identify the sources of protein as
   either animal or plant.   *6 points*

Food containing Protein	Source

9. List three reasons why we need
    lipids in the body   *3 points*
    a. _____
    b. _____
    c. _____
10. What are lipids?   *2 points*
    _____

LESSON FOUR

OVERVIEW OF NUTRITION—PART IV
VITAMINS

Age level: 10-15 years   **Class time**: 50 minutes

Teaching Objectives

The objectives of this lesson are to:

- ◈ Differentiate between the two groups of vitamins essential for good health
- ◈ Discuss the roles of vitamins in the body
- ◈ Identify food sources of vitamins

Learning Outcomes

By the end of the lesson, students should be able to:

- ◈ Name four fat-soluble and two water-soluble vitamins
- ◈ Describe a role that each vitamin plays in the body
- ◈ Name food sources of each vitamin

Materials Needed: pictures of food items (vegetables and fruits) and letter cards spelling out the word vitamins

Introduction

Time allocated: 5 minutes

Teaching method: Activity and lecture

Teaching activity:

Teacher distributes letter cards to students, which spell out the word—**V I T A M I N S**. Their task is to make a word. Please, make it quickly. *"Vitamins"* You have probably heard a lot about vitamins. Maybe you take vitamin pills or hear adults tell you to eat your vegetables because they are loaded with vitamins. But what exactly are vitamins?

40

Section A: Identification of Vitamins

Time allocated: 10 minutes

Summary

Vitamins are found in many foods and they do not supply energy as carbohydrates, fats and proteins do, but they are essential because they **regulate the body chemistry and body functions.** Vitamins cannot be produced by our bodies. They must be eaten in our food. Vitamins assist the body in using food by bringing about biochemical reactions so life can be maintained.

Vitamins are divided into two groups. The first group, **fat-soluble vitamins** are usually stored in your body until you need them. The second group, **water-soluble vitamins**, travels through your bloodstream, and are either used right away or sent out of your body when you urinate. All vitamins have special jobs to do in your body. Table 4.1 lists the vitamins essential for good health. More vitamins have been identified, but their contributions to good health have not been established.

Table 4.1. Vitamins needed for good health

Fat-soluble Vitamins	Water-soluble Vitamins
Vitamin A	Vitamin C (ascorbic acid)
Vitamin D	Vitamin B_1 (thiamin)
Vitamin E	Vitamin B_2 (riboflavin)
Vitamin K	Vitamin B_3 (niacin)
	Vitamin B_6 (pyridoxine)
	Vitamin B_{12} (cobalamin)
	Folacin (Folate or Folic acid)

Section B: Functions of Vitamins

Time allocated: 10 minutes

Teaching method: Lecture

Teaching activity:

◈ Explain to students the functions of vitamins

Summary

Function of Vitamins

FAT-SOLUBLE VITAMINS

Vitamin A

◈ Vital to good vision
◈ Prevents night blindness
◈ Necessary for healthy skin, hair growth
◈ Keeps mucous membranes healthy
◈ Severe deficiency causes blindness

Vitamin D

◈ Helps bones use the mineral calcium to build strong bones
◈ Prevents rickets

Vitamin E

◈ Helps break down polyunsaturated fats
◈ Protects blood cell membranes from overexposure to oxygen

Vitamin K

◈ Essential for clotting of blood

WATER-SOLUBLE VITAMINS

Vitamin C

- Also called ascorbic acid
- Helps form collagen or body cement
- Helps in growth and repair of body tissue and blood vessels
- Prevents scurvy

Vitamin B Group

B_1-Thiamine

- Energy metabolism, nerve function and muscle control

B_2-Riboflavin

- Involved in use of fat, protein and carbohydrates

B_3-Niacin

- Energy metabolism, maintain healthy nervous system and skin

B_6-Pyridoxine

- Normal immune and nervous system

B_{12}-Cobalamin

- Produces antibodies, helps folacin function, maintenance of nerve tissue

Folacin

- Synthesise DNA; cell division

Section C: Food Sources of Vitamins

Time allocated: 10 minutes

Teaching method: Class discussion

Summary:

Food Sources of Vitamins

Fat-Soluble Vitamins			
Vitamin A	**Vitamin D**	**Vitamin E**	**Vitamin K**
Meats, liver, crab, eggs, milk and milk products, butter, margarine *Beta-carotene* —mango, pumpkin, sweet potato, carrot, watermelon, spinach, paw-paw, sweet pepper, tomato, broccoli, orange, greens	Milk, fish and seafood, salmon, tuna, shrimp, liver, egg yolk, sunlight	Oil, margarine, peanuts, cashew nuts, sweet potato, greens, spinach, wheat germ, bread, crab, shrimp, fish	Greens, beef broccoli, liver cabbage, spinach

Water-Soluble Vitamins			
Vitamin B$_1$	**Vitamin B$_2$**	**Niacin**	**Vitamin B$_6$**
Meats, peanuts, brown rice, macaroni, bread, peas, corn, orange, peas, broccoli, avocado, greens, pork	Milk and milk products, meats, tuna fish, greens, broccoli, eggs, macaroni, bread	Meats, tuna fish, poultry, peanuts, vegetables, rice, milk and milk products	Salmon, other fish, poultry, eggs, peas and beans, banana, greens, liver, avocado, carrots, sweet potato
Vitamin B$_{12}$	**Folacin**	**Vitamin C**	
Liver, beef, lamb, crab, tuna, veal, hamburger, milk and milk products, eggs	Vegetables, Black-eyed peas, spinach, beans, peas, orange, oatmeal, wild rice, wheat germ	Citrus fruits, sweet peppers, greens, tomatoes, watermelon, broccoli	

Evaluation (see next page)

Time allocated: 10 minutes

Assignment: List ten food sources/examples for: a) Fat-soluble vitamins; b) Water-soluble vitamins

Instruction: assignment should be handed in at the next lesson

Closure   *Time allocated*: 5 minutes

Teaching activity: Teacher summarises the lesson and invites questions from students.

EVALUATION—OVERVIEW OF NUTRITION—PART IV
VITAMINS

Name: _____   Maximum points: 10

Instructions: For your evaluation, you will be given a vitamin to advertise. In your advertisement, you must include the following information:

The name of the vitamin

All the FUNCTIONS of the vitamin

List at least two FOOD SOURCES of the vitamin

Name the deficiency disease caused by lack or insufficient amounts of the vitamin

You will be graded according to the following:

VITAMIN

TOPICS COVERED:

NAME OR IDENTIFICATION	1	2	3	4	5
FOOD SOURCES	1	2	3	4	5
FUNCTIONS	1	2	3	4	5
DEFICIENCY	1	2	3	4	5
CREATIVITY	1	2	3	4	5
USE OF TIME AND PRESENTATION	1	2	3	4	5

TOTAL POINTS EARNED

LESSON FIVE

OVERVIEW OF NUTRITION—PART V
MINERALS

Age level: 10-15 years   **Class time**: 50 minutes

Teaching Objectives

The objectives of this lesson are to:

◆ Identify the macro—and trace—minerals essential for good health

◆ Discuss the roles of minerals in the body

◆ Identify food sources of minerals

Learning Outcomes

By the end of the lesson, students should be able to:

◆ Identify and name the macro—and trace—minerals

◆ Describe a role that each mineral plays in the body

◆ Name food sources of each mineral

Materials Needed: pictures of food items; vegetables; fruits; text about vitamins; diagram about vitamins, where they are found, what they are useful for, how they are used, and what happens when someone is deficient; letter cards spelling out the word vitamins

Introduction

Time allocated: 5 minutes

Teaching method: Discussion, lecture and activity

Teaching activity:

Ask students to come to the teacher. Teacher gives them letter cards, which spell out: M I N E R A L S. Their task is to make a word. Please, make it quickly. "Minerals"
You have probably heard about minerals, but what exactly

are minerals? Students answer, then teacher gets into the lesson.

Section A: Identification of Minerals

Time allocated: 10 minutes

Summary

Minerals are found in nearly all the foods listed in the Six Basic Food Groups of the Caribbean. They do not supply energy as carbohydrates, fats and proteins do, but they are essential because they **regulate the body chemistry and body functions**.

Minerals cannot be produced by our bodies. They must be eaten in our food. Minerals are also found in enzymes, hormones, bones and muscles. Minerals can become part of the body's structure. There are about 60 different minerals that make up about 4% of the body. Science is still learning about many of the functions of minerals. Minerals are divided into two groups: i) **Macro-minerals** are found in relatively large amounts; and ii) **trace-minerals**, which are found in very small amounts in the body. Table 5.1. shows the minerals needed for good health.

Table 5.1 Minerals Needed for Good Health

MACRO-MINERALS	TRACE-MINERALS
Calcium	Iron
Phosphorus	Zinc
Sodium	Fluorine
Potassium	Copper
	Iodine

Section B: Functions of Minerals

Time allocated: 15 minutes

Teaching method: Lecture

Teaching activity:

◆ Explain to students the functions of minerals

Summary

Functions of Minerals

MINERAL	FUNCTION
Macro-minerals	
Calcium	Bones, teeth, blood clotting, aids heart and nervous system
Phosphorus	Works with calcium; releases energy
Sodium	Regulates fluid, muscles, heart, nerves
Potassium	Regulates fluid, muscles, heart, nerves
Trace-minerals	
Iron	Blood-hemoglobin, carries oxygen to cells
Zinc	Growth, maintenance of body
Fluorine	Teeth and bones, works with calcium
Copper	Red blood cells
Iodine	Thyroid
"Fibre"	Aids the digestive system, cannot be digested

Summary:

Food Sources of Minerals

Macrominerals

Calcium	Sodium	Potassium	Phosphorous
Milk and milk products, Spinach, broccoli, greens, dried beans, Lima beans	Salt, processed foods, corned beef, meatloaf, sausage, hot dog, smoked fish, corned fish, salted fish, soy sauce	Vegetables, tomato, celery, carrots, broccoli, avocado, banana, orange juice watermelon, raisins, prunes, meats, fish, grains, milk and milk products, salt substitutes	Milk and milk products, meats, nuts and seeds, grains, potato, corn, peas, broccoli

Trace-minerals

Iron	Zinc	Iodine
Meat and dried beans, grains, prune juice, raisins, plums, spinach	Meats, dried peas and beans, grains, nuts and seeds, milk and milk products	Seafoods, iodised salt

Evaluation (see next page)

Time allocated: 10 minutes

Assignment: List ten food sources/examples for:

    a) Macro-minerals

    b) Trace-minerals

Instruction: assignment should be handed in at the next lesson

Closure

Time allocated: 10 minutes

Teaching activity: Teacher summarises the lesson and invites questions from students.

EVALUATION—OVERVIEW OF NUTRITION—PART IV
MINERALS

Name: _____   Maximum points: 10

Instructions: Make a similar table and fill in the functions
and food sources of the minerals, we studied.

MINERAL	FUNCTION	SOURCES
Calcium		
Phosphorus		
Potassium		
Sodium		
Iron		
Zinc		

LESSON FIVE - EVALUATION

Iodine		
"Fibre," also called Roughage Cellulose		

WATER

The human body is anywhere from 55 to 78% water depending on body size. Water is the main component of human body. The body's tissues and organs are mainly made up of water—a breakdown follows:

◈ Muscles—75% water
◈ Brain—75-90% water
◈ Bone—22% water
◈ Blood—83-92% water

The functions of water in the human body are vital as shown in Figure 5.1.

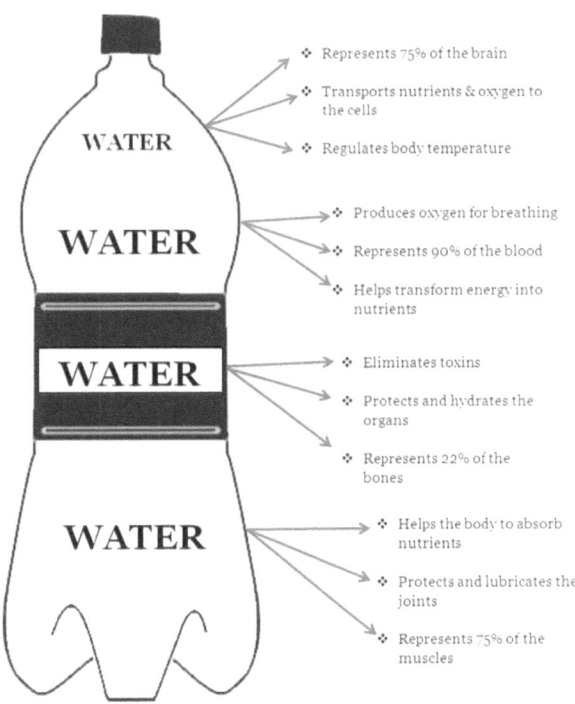

❖ Represents 75% of the brain
❖ Transports nutrients & oxygen to the cells
❖ Regulates body temperature
❖ Produces oxygen for breathing
❖ Represents 90% of the blood
❖ Helps transform energy into nutrients
❖ Eliminates toxins
❖ Protects and hydrates the organs
❖ Represents 22% of the bones
❖ Helps the body to absorb nutrients
❖ Protects and lubricates the joints
❖ Represents 75% of the muscles

Figure 5.1. Functions of Water in the Human Body

LESSON SIX

CARBOHYDRATE DIGESTION

Age level: 10-15 years   **Class time**: 45 minutes

Teaching Objectives

The objectives of this lesson are to:

- ◈ Define digestion
- ◈ Discuss the process involved in carbohydrate digestion
- ◈ Identify the end product of carbohydrate digestion
- ◈ Discuss insulin and its role in carbohydrate digestion

Learning Outcomes

By the end of the lesson, students should be able to:

- ◈ Define digestion
- ◈ Discuss digestion of carbohydrates
- ◈ Identify the end product of carbohydrate digestion
- ◈ Discuss insulin and its role in carbohydrate digestion

Relevant Previous Knowledge

- • Overview of Nutrition

Materials Needed

- • Diagram on digestive system (Figure 6.1.)
- • Keys

Introduction

Time allocated: 2 minutes

Teaching method: Lecture

Summary:

When food is eaten, it is broken down into smaller forms so that the body can make use of the nutrients, which helps us to produce energy, repair worn out tissues and protect the body against diseases.

Section A—Definition of Digestion

Time Allocated: 10 minutes

Teaching method: Discussion

Teacher's activity:

- ◈ Ask students *"what is digestion?"*
- ◈ Explain briefly the meaning of digestion (see summary) using Figure 6.1. to illustrate

Summary:

Digestion

Our digestive (say: dye-jes-tiv) systems starts working even before we take the first bite of our bread. The digestive system will be busy at work on your chewed-up lunch for the next few hours—or sometimes days, depending upon what you have eaten. This process, called **digestion**, allows your body to get the nutrients and energy it needs from the food you eat.

The human digestive system processes food that we eat. It is made up of many organs and glands that digest the food, extract energy and nutrients, and later excrete the waste by-product.

The digestive system has two major parts:

I. Upper gastrointestinal tract

II. Lower gastrointestinal tract

The **upper gastrointestinal (GI) tract** comprises mainly of the mouth, pharynx, oesophagus and stomach, while the lower **gastrointestinal (GI) tract** consists of the small intestine, large intestine and anus. Organs such as the liver, gallbladder and pancreas are also parts of the digestive system.

Section B—Digestion of Carbohydrate

Time allocated: 10 minutes

Teaching method: Class discussion

Sample questions: Ask students to observe the digestive system critically.

Teacher's activity:

◈ Explain to students how food is digested from the mouth down to the small intestines and emphasise the organs involved in the process.

◈ Point out the following organs on Figure 6.1 and explain to students how they work to digest carbohydrates: mouth, pancreas, gallbladder, small intestine, large intestine and anus

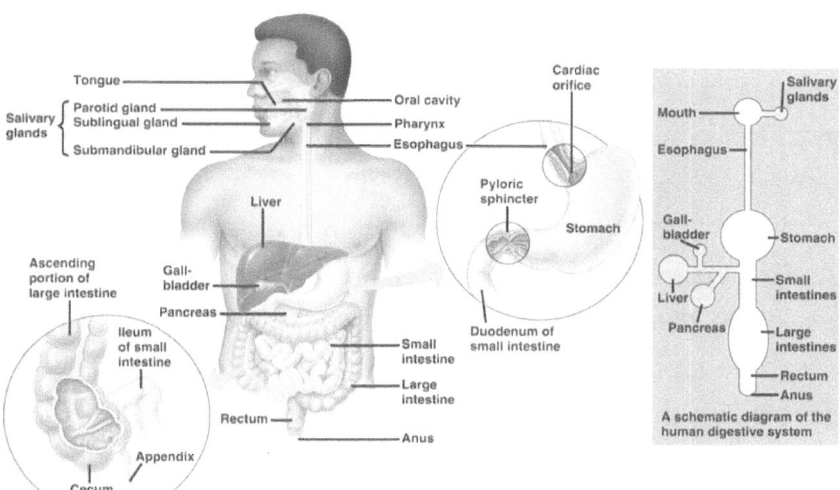

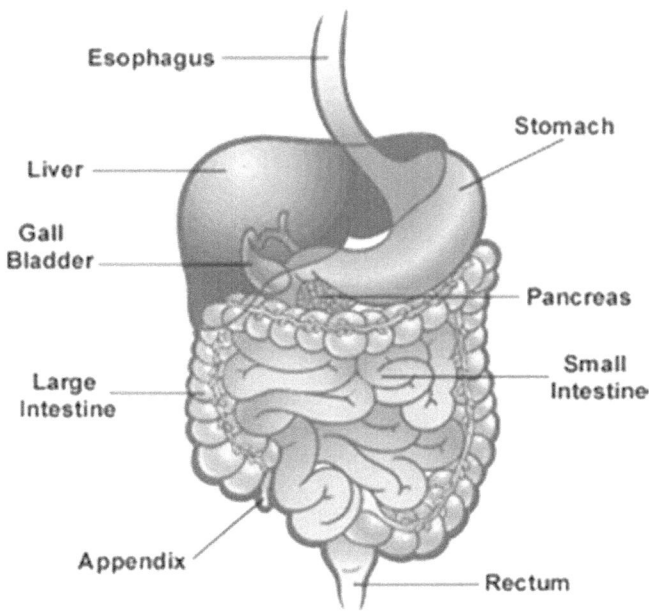

Figure 6.1. The Human Digestive System

Source: http://poster.4teachers.org

Summary

Digestion of Carbohydrates

First, food enters the body via the **mouth**, where saliva from the **salivary glands** begins to break down carbohydrates into glucose with the help of **enzymes** in the mouth. **Enzymes are living organisms that speed up processes in the body.** Examples of carbohydrate foods includes: bread, potatoes, yams etc. (Lesson one). Next, the food goes down the food tube, the **oesophagus** pushed by muscular contractions. The food ends up in the stomach. The liver processes and regulates the substances entering the blood stream from the food that is consumed. The liver also produces **bile**, which is stored in the **gall bladder**. The bile breaks down fat and kills germs and bacteria present in the food.

The **pancreas,** an organ near the stomach, assists in digestion of carbohydrates; it produces a hormone called **insulin,** which regulates blood sugar levels by directing cells to take up or to secrete sugar into the blood. Once food leaves the stomach, it travels to the **small intestines** where carbohydrates are absorbed.

Absorption is the uptake of nutrients into or across tissues in the body. After entering the **large intestine**, moisture is absorbed from what is left of the food, and bacteria break down some of the materials, which have not been digested. This creates waste (**faeces**). The **rectum** is the final storage space for waste, which is what becomes of the food once all of the nutrients and moisture have been removed. The waste remains in the rectum until excreted.

Section C: End—Product of Carbohydrate Digestion

Time allocated: 2 minutes

Teaching method: Brainstorming

Teacher's activity: Teacher brainstorms students on the end-product of digestion

[Sample question: *what do you think the breakdown of carbohydrates will be?]*

Summary

The end product of carbohydrates is **glucose**. Glucose provides our body with energy.

Section D: Insulin: Role in Carbohydrate Digestion

Time allocated: 5 minutes

Teaching method: Discussion and Demonstration

Teacher's activity

Illustrate how insulin works by using a key to open the classroom door and explain to students how the insulin opens the cells and muscles up for uptake of glucose.

Summary

Carbohydrates are broken down to **glucose** in the small intestines and then absorbed into the bloodstream. Glucose cannot enter fat or muscle cells because glucose channels are closed—so glucose cannot be burned for energy in the cells.

The pancreas detects an increase in glucose levels in the bloodstream and pumps **insulin** into the bloodstream. **Insulin** unlocks the cells' glucose channels so the muscles and cells can take up glucose through the open channels. The glucose level in the bloodstream falls as glucose is taken up by the cells and muscles. The **pancreas** detects the falling blood glucose level and switches off secretion of insulin.

Glucose is burned up for energy in the body cells.

Evaluation: See next page

Time allocated: 10 minutes

Closure

Time allocated: 5 minutes

Activity: Teacher summarises the lesson and invites questions from students.

Assignment: Draw and label the human digestive system.

EVALUATION—CARBOHYDRATE DIGESTION

Name: _____   Maximum Points: 10

Answer all Questions Correctly

Circle True or False for the sentences below.

1. Digestion allows our bodies to get the
    nutrients and energy it needs from the
    food we eat.   . . . True   . . . False   *1 point*
2. Glucose is the main fuel
    for the body.   . . . True   . . . False   *1 point*

Fill in the blanks using the given words

3. Carbohydrate digestions begin in the . . .
    a. Nose   b. stomach   c. mouth   *1 point*
4. Glucose is the end product of . . .
    a. Carbohydrates   b. fat   c. protein   *2 points*

Match the following pairs:

Mouth	Insulin
Liver	Salivary gland
Pancreas	Gall bladder
Small intestines	Excretion
Rectum	Absorption *5 points*

OVERVIEW OF DIABETES

Age level: 10-15 years   **Class time**: 45 minutes

Teaching Objectives

The objectives of this lesson are to:

◆ Define diabetes

◆ Identify common symptoms of diabetes

◆ Explain the difference between the types of diabetes

Learning Outcomes

By the end of the lesson students should be able to:

◆ Define diabetes

◆ Identify five symptoms of diabetes

◆ Differentiate between the types of diabetes

Relevant Previous Knowledge:

◆ Overview of Nutrition

◆ Carbohydrate Digestion

Materials Needed

◆ Pictures on each symptom of diabetes (Figures 7.1-7.7)

◆ Digestion pathways of people without diabetes, people with type I and people with type II diabetes (Figures 7.8-7.10)

Introduction

Time: 3 minutes

Teaching method: Brainstorming

Teaching activity: Recap the lesson on carbohydrate digestion.

Sample questions

◈ *Which foods contain carbohydrates?*

◈ *What is the end-product of carbohydrate breakdown?*

◈ *What is insulin?*

Section A: Definition of Diabetes

Time: 5 minutes

Teaching method: Discussion and Lecture

Teacher's Activity: Ask students what they know about diabetes

Summary

Diabetes is a disease that affects how the body uses food for energy or as fuel. When the body's cells cannot use food properly, the blood glucose or sugar becomes high. **Glucose** comes from the digestion of starchy foods such as bread, rice, potatoes, yams, sugars and other sweet foods (previous lessons). The blood glucose becomes higher, either because the body lacks insulin or because it cannot use the insulin it makes.

Recap on Insulin: a hormone produced by the pancreas, which helps glucose get into the cells for energy. Diabetes is not caused by eating sweets.

Section B: Symptoms of Diabetes

Time: 7 minutes

Teaching method: Class discussion.

Materials needed: Pictures on each symptom of diabetes; digestive systems of people without diabetes and those with types 1 and 2 diabetes

Teaching Activity: Ask students to observe and describe what is happening in each picture.

Summary

Symptoms of Diabetes

◆ Frequent urination

◆ Thirst

◆ Dizziness

◆ Blurred vision

◆ Weight loss

◆ Excessive hunger

◆ Irritability

Section C—Types of Diabetes

Time: 10 minutes

Teaching method: Group discussion

Materials needed: Digestive system on people without diabetes, type 1 and type 2 diabetes (Figure 7.2. a, b, c)

Teaching Activity: Divide students into three groups

• Group A—students without diabetes (Figure 7.2 a)

• Group B—students with type I diabetes (Figure 7.2 b)

• Group C—students with type II diabetes (Figure 7.2 c)

Sample questions:

• *Group A identifies and discusses what is seen on (Figure 7.2 a)*

• *Group B identifies and discusses what is seen on (Figure 7.2 b)*

• *Group C identifies and discusses what is seen on (Figure 7.2 c)*

Teaching activity: Explain to each group (using the Figures), the importance of insulin.

Summary

Type 1 diabetes develops when the insulin-producing cells in the body have been destroyed, and the body is unable to produce any insulin. Insulin is the key that unlocks the door to the body's cells. Once the door is unlocked, glucose can enter the cells where it is used as fuel. In Type 1 diabetes the body is unable to produce any insulin so there is no key to unlock the door and the glucose builds up in the blood (Figure 7.2. b).

Nobody knows for sure why these insulin-producing cells have been destroyed, but the most likely cause is the body having an abnormal reaction to the cells. This may be triggered by a virus or other infection. Type 1 diabetes can develop at any age but usually appears before the age of 40, and especially in childhood. Type 1 diabetes accounts for between 5 and 15% of all people with diabetes and is treated by daily insulin injections, a healthy diet and regular physical activity.

Type 2 diabetes develops when the body can still make some insulin, but not enough, or when the insulin that is produced does not work properly (known as **insulin resistance**). Insulin acts as a key unlocking the cells, so if there is not enough insulin, or it is not working properly, the cells are only partially unlocked (or not at all) and glucose builds up in the blood (Figure 7.2 c).

Type 2 diabetes usually appears in people over the age of 40, though in South Asian and people of African descent, who are at greater risk, it often appears from the age of 25. It is also increasingly becoming more common in children, adolescents and young people of all ethnicities. Type 2 diabetes accounts for between 85 and 95% of all people with diabetes and is treated with a healthy diet and increased physical activity. In addition to this, medication and/or insulin are often required.

Some risk factors for type 2 diabetes include:

Family history

Overweight

Unhealthy diet

Lack of exercise

Evaluation: (see next page)
Time allocated: 10 minutes
Assignment: Describe four symptoms of diabetes
Closure:
Time allocated: 10 minutes
Teaching activity: Teacher summarises the main points of the lesson and invites questions from students.

EVALUATION—OVERVIEW OF DIABETES

Name: _____   Maximum Points: 15

Answer all Questions Correctly

Circle True or False for the sentences below.

1. Glucose comes from digestion
   of carbohydrates.   . . . True   . . . False   *1 point*
2. Type I diabetes usually occurs
   in children.   . . . True   . . . False   *1 point*
3. Type II diabetes is cause by
   eating sweets.   . . . True   . . . False   *1 point*
4. All overweight people will
   get diabetes.   . . . True   . . . False   *1 point*
5. Diabetes is a disease that involves
   blood sugar levels.   . . . True   . . . False   *1 point*
6. Healthy eating is one treatment for
   type 2 diabetes.   . . . True   . . . False   *1 point*

Fill in the blanks

7. Diabetes is a disease that affects the body's use of . . . *1 point*
   a. Water   b. Glucose   c. Vitamins
8. Glucose is used by the body and turned into . . .   *1 point*
   a. Energy   b. Starch   c. Carbohydrates
9. The pancreas makes a hormone called . . .   *1 point*
   a. Growth hormone   b. Insulin   c. Thyroid hormone

10. Lemons are to oranges as sugar is to . . .   *1 point*
    a. Hormones   b. Salt   c. Glucose   d. Juice

11. List 5 symptoms of diabetes.   *5 points*
    _____
    _____
    _____
    _____
    _____

Symptoms of Diabetes

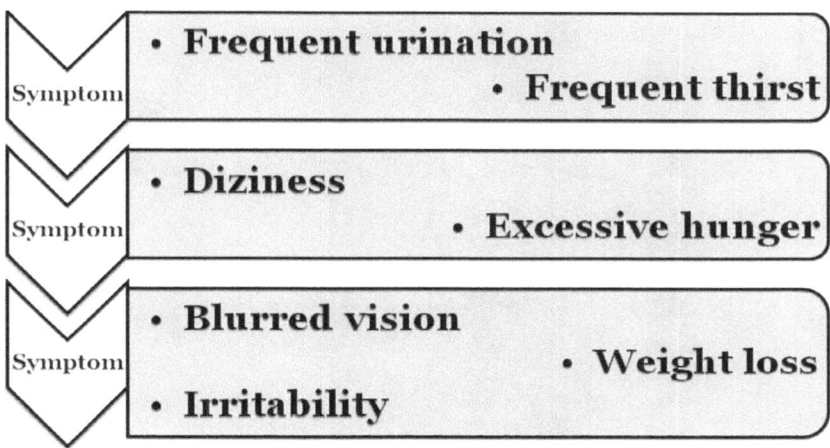

Figure 7. Symptoms of Diabetes

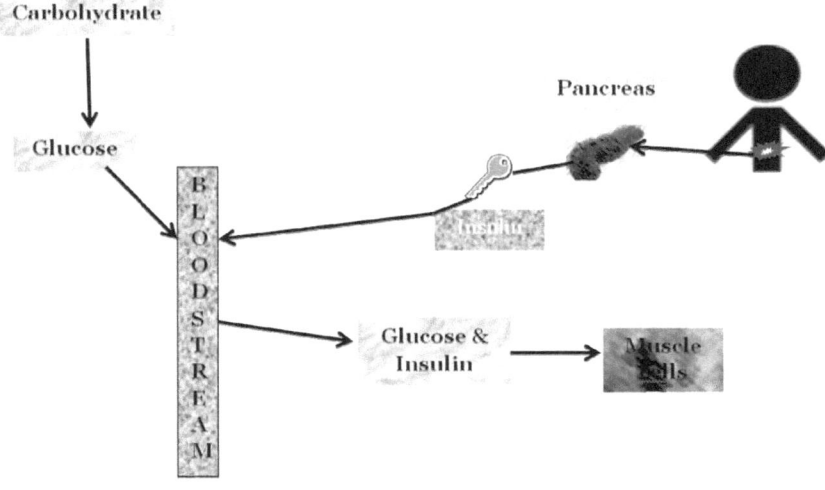

Figure 7.2a. People without Diabetes

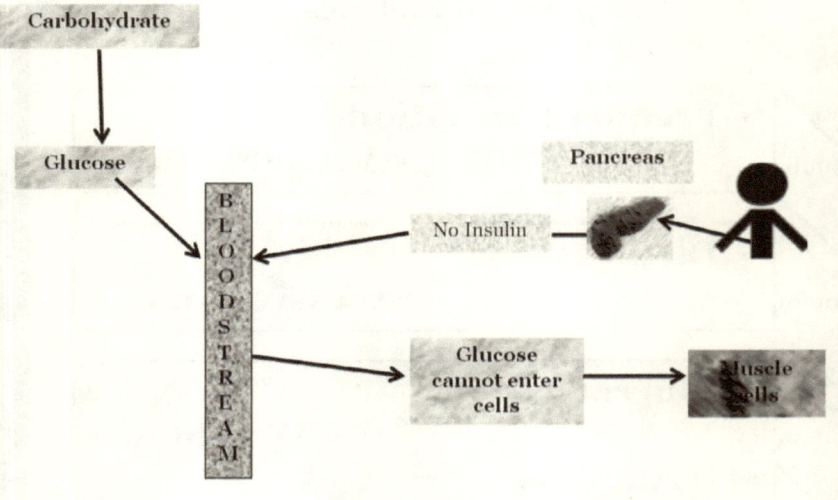

Figure 7.2b. People with Type 1 Diabetes

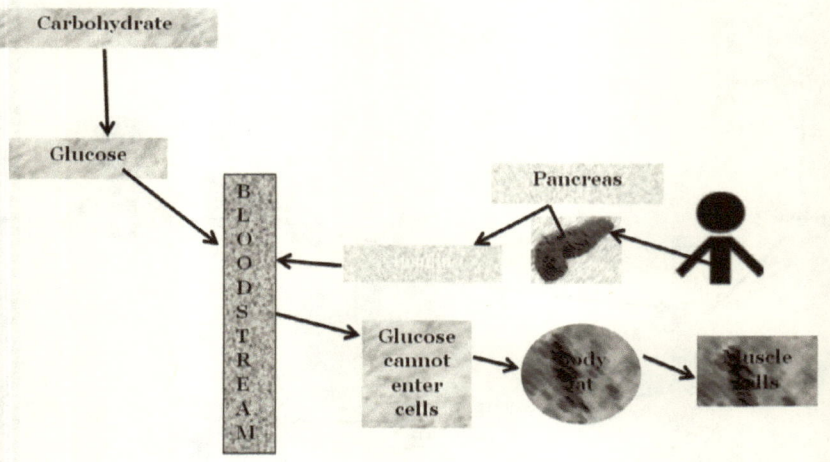

Figure 7.2c. People with Type 2 Diabetes

LESSON EIGHT

COMPLICATIONS IN DIABETES

Age level: 10-15 years   **Class time**: 45 minutes

Teaching Objectives

The objectives of this lesson are to:

- ◈ Define hypoglycemia and hyperglycemia
- ◈ State causes of hypoglycemia and hyperglycemia
- ◈ Sate symptoms of hyperglycemia and hypoglycemia

Learning Outcomes

By the end of the lesson students should be able to:

- ◈ Define hypoglycemia and hyperglycemia
- ◈ List causes of hypo—and hyperglycemia
- ◈ State symptoms of hypo—and hyperglycemia

Relevant previous knowledge

- ◈ Overview of Nutrition
- ◈ Carbohydrate Digestion
- ◈ Overview of Diabetes

Introduction

Time allocated: 2 minutes

Teaching activity: Recall on the role of insulin in carbohydrate digestion

Section A: Definition of Hypoglycemia

Time allocated: 3 minutes

Teaching method: Lecture

Summary

Blood Sugar Levels

Before meals or upon waking	2 hours after the start of a meal
A person with Type 2 diabetes	
70-130 mg/dL	< 180 mg/dL; (less than 180 mg/dL)
A person without diabetes	
83 mg/dL or less	<120 mg/dL; (less than 120 mg/dL)

Hypoglycemia is a condition characterized by an abnormally low level of blood sugar (glucose), your body's main energy source. Immediate treatment of hypoglycemia involves quick steps to get your blood sugar level back into a normal range, either with high-sugar foods or medications.

Section B—Causes of Hypoglycemia

Time allocated: 3 minutes

Teaching method: Brainstorming

Brainstorming question

Since we get glucose from the food we eat, what are some factors that would cause a fall in blood glucose level?

Summary

Causes of hypoglycemia include:

- ◈ Eating too little food
- ◈ Delaying a meal
- ◈ Doing more exercise than you normally do
- ◈ Missing a meal
- ◈ Taking too much diabetes medicine

Section C: Symptoms of Hypoglycemia

Time allocated: 5 minutes

Teaching method: Questions and answers

Sample question:

- ◈ *What happens to the body when it has no energy?*
- ◈ *How do you feel when you are hungry?*

Summary

Most people with hypoglycemia have the following signs or symptoms

- ◈ Rapid heart beat
- ◈ Confusion
- ◈ Shakiness
- ◈ Anger
- ◈ Sweating
- ◈ Fainting

Section D: Definition of Hyperglycemia

Time allocated: 3 minutes

Teacher's activity: Lecture

Summary

Hyperglycemia is the technical term for high blood glucose (sugar). High blood glucose happens when the body has too little insulin or when the body cannot use insulin properly.

Section E: Causes of Hyperglycemia

Time allocated: 5 minutes

Teaching method: Brainstorming

Sample question

Since the body is unable to use glucose, what are some factors that can cause a rise in blood glucose levels?

Summary

The following can lead to increased in blood sugar level:

◆ Eating foods containing too many carbohydrates

◆ Not producing enough insulin action either by injection of insulin or by medicine

◆ Stress can also play a role in causing hyperglycemia

◆ Low levels of exercise. Daily exercise is a critical contributor to regulating blood sugar levels.

◆ With illness, blood glucose tends to rise rapidly

Section F: Symptoms of Hyperglycemia

Time allocated: 3 minutes

Teaching method: Lecture

Summary

Symptoms of hyperglycemia include:

◆ Drowsiness

◆ Very dry mouth and body tissue

◆ Inability to speak

◆ Weakness of parts of the body

◆ Fainting or becoming unconscious

◆ Hallucinations

Evaluation: (see next page)

Time allocated: 10 minutes

Assignment: List five causes and symptoms of hyperglycemia and five ways of treating hyperglycemia.

Closure

Time allocated: 10 minutes

Teacher summarises the main points of the lesson, and invites questions from students.

EVALUATION—COMPLICATIONS IN DIABETES

Name: _____   Maximum Points: 15

Answer all Questions Correctly

Circle True or False for the sentences below.

1. Hypoglycemia is high
   blood sugar.   . . . True   . . . False   *1 point*
2. Hyperglycemia is high
   blood sugar.   . . . True   . . . False   *1 point*

Instructions: Check the correct answer(s)   *9 points*

3. Hypoglycemia can be caused by:
   . . . Eating too little food
   . . . Talking to a friend
   . . . Delaying a meal
   . . . Doing more exercise than you normally do
4. Hyperglycemia can be caused by:
   . . . Eating foods containing too much carbohydrates
   . . . Infections
   . . . Talking in class
   . . . Not producing enough insulin
5. The following are symptoms of
   hypoglycemia **EXCEPT**   *2 points*
      a. Anger   b. Sweating   c. Shakiness   d. Salivating
6. The following are symptoms of
   hyperglycemia **EXCEPT**
      a. Inability to speak. b. Drowsiness c. Dry mouth
      d. Dry throat   *2 points*

LESSON NINE

DIABETES PREVENTION AND CONTROL—HEALTHY EATING

Age level: 10-15 years   **Class time**: 45 minutes

Teaching Objectives

The objectives of this lesson are to:

Define the following terms: calories, serving size and percentage daily value (%DV)

- ◆ View PowerPoint presentation on the Caribbean Food Groups
- ◆ Describe the six Caribbean Food Groups
- ◆ List the guidelines for healthy food choices
- ◆ Read food labels

Learning Outcomes

By the end of the lesson, students should be able to:

- ◆ Define calories; serving size; and percent daily value (% DV)
- ◆ Create a chart showing the Caribbean Food Groups using the foods shown, along with other foods that they like to eat
- ◆ List three guidelines for healthy food choices
- ◆ Accurately read food labels

Relevant previous knowledge

- ◆ Overview of Nutrition
- ◆ Carbohydrate Digestion
- ◆ Overview of Diabetes
- ◆ Complications in Diabetes

Materials needed:
- ◈ Food pictures, coloring pencils, ruler
- ◈ Sample food label (Figure 9.1.)
- ◈ Ask students to bring food labels of their favourite snacks to class

Section A—Definition of Terms

Time allocated: 5 minutes

Teaching methods: Lecture

Summary

Definition of terms

- ◈ **A calorie** is a unit of heat used to express the energy value of food. One pound of fat stores about **3,500 calories** so, in order to lose a pound of fat, you need to burn an extra 3,500 calories. To lose a pound in one week, that would mean creating a calorie deficit of 500 calories per day with diet, exercise or both. Calories are supplied by carbohydrates (sugars and starch), fats and proteins as we learnt earlier.

- ◈ **A serving size** is a referenced amount of food that allows you to compare the nutritional value of different foods. The serving size also functions as a portion control mechanism. Serving sizes can help you determine how much and what type of foods to eat. The Caribbean Food Groups and the nutritional facts label use the concept of serving size to facilitate the nutritional and caloric comparisons of similar foods. The serving size for a particular food, however, may differ between the Caribbean Food Groups and the nutrition facts panel of the label.

◈ **The Percent Daily Value (%DV)** on the Nutrition Facts Panel of a food label is a number that tells you if there is a lot or a little of a nutrient (like calcium) in one serving of food. % DV puts nutrients on a scale from 0% to 100%.

◈ *What is a little and what is a lot?* For example, 5% DV or less of a nutrient is considered low because it is low on the scale; 20% DV or more is high. If the label says, *"Calcium 4%"*, that means one serving of the food has 4% of the calcium that a person needs in one day. However, note that: (a) the percentage is calculated for an adult who needs 1,000 milligrams of calcium per day and (b) children need more calcium than most adults.

  o Again, if a nutrient has 5 % of the daily value or less, it is low in that nutrient. This can be good or bad depending on if it is a nutrient you want more or less of.

  o If it has 20% or more, it is higher in that nutrient, this can be good for nutrients like fibre or nutrients you want to get more of, but not so good for something like saturated fat (a nutrient you need less of).

Section B: Creating a Chart of the Caribbean Food Groups

Time allocated: 5 minutes

Teaching method: Class discussion and illustration.

Teaching activity: distribute paper plate and coloring pencils to each student in the class.

Summary

o Using the plates, students will sort and group the food pictures according to their similarity and/or differences. Create a name for each group you have identified and write down the names of other foods that they eat in each category.

o Have students view PowerPoint presentation on the *"Caribbean Food Groups"* as teacher explains the groups. To maintain healthy eating habits and to have a balanced diet, it is important to utilise these food groups with special emphasis on the healthier options within each group. The daily intake of food for all humans should be proportionately represented as in the plate, with **the largest percentage from the staples group** and **the smallest amount from the fats and oils group.** A balanced diet is one comprising foods from all the six food groups in adequate quantities to provide all essential nutrients.

o Students will then create a poster labelled the *"Caribbean Food Groups"*

NB: this strategy will help you eat fewer calories and feel fuller.

The Caribbean Food Groups—A Guide to Meal Planning for Healthy Eating

Source: Caribbean Food and Nutrition Institute. The six food groups; available at:

http://www.paho.org/cfni/index.php; accessed 9/25/2013

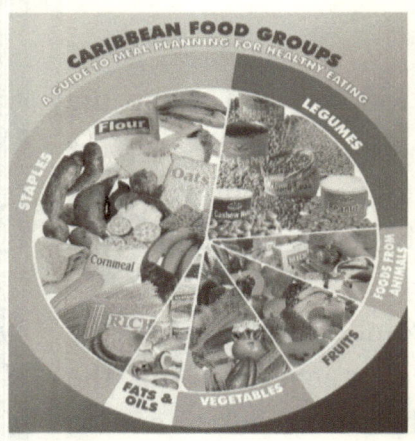

Powerpoint Presentation

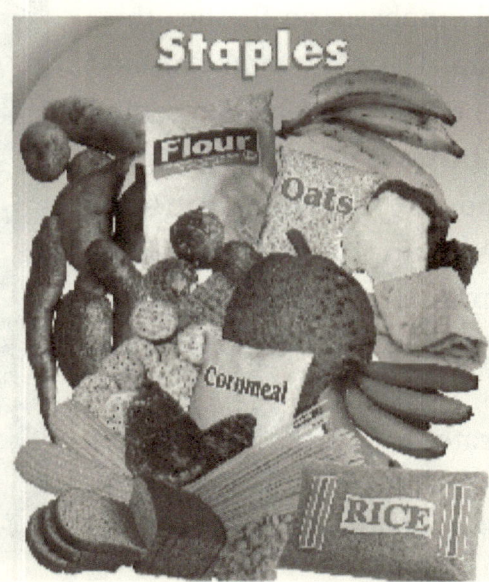

Cereals:
Bread (from whole grain or enriched flour), wheat flour, corn (maize), cornmeal, dried cereals, macaroni, spaghetti, rice, cereal porridges.

Starchy fruits, roots, tubers/ground provisions: Banana, plantain, breadfruit, yam, potato, dasheen, coco/eddoe, cassava.

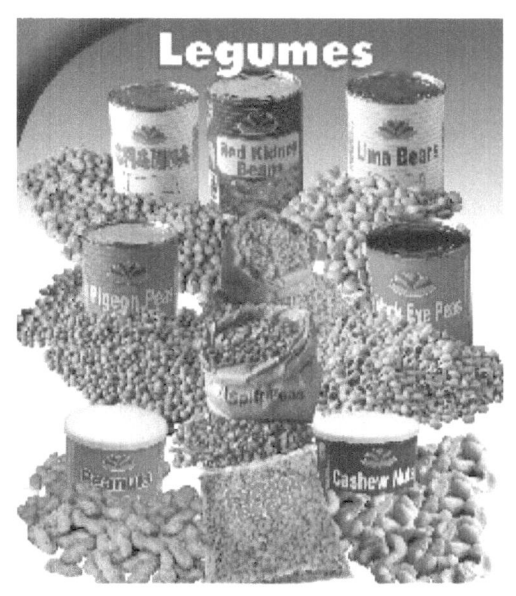

Kidney beans, gungo/pigeon peas, black-eye peas, cow peas, other dried peas and beans, peanuts, cashew nuts, sesame seeds, pumpkin seeds.

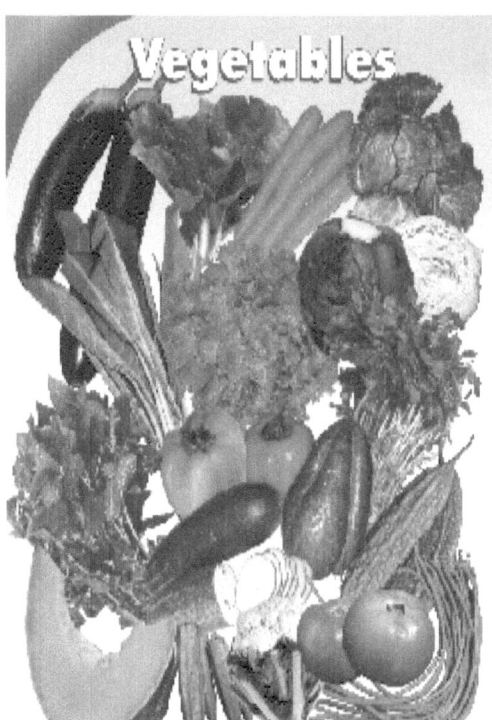

Dark green leafy and yellow vegetables:
Callaloo/spinach, dasheen leaves, cabbage bush, pak choy, string beans, pumpkin, carrot.

Other vegetables:
Squash, cho-cho, (christophene, chayote), cucumber, tomato, garden egg/aubergine

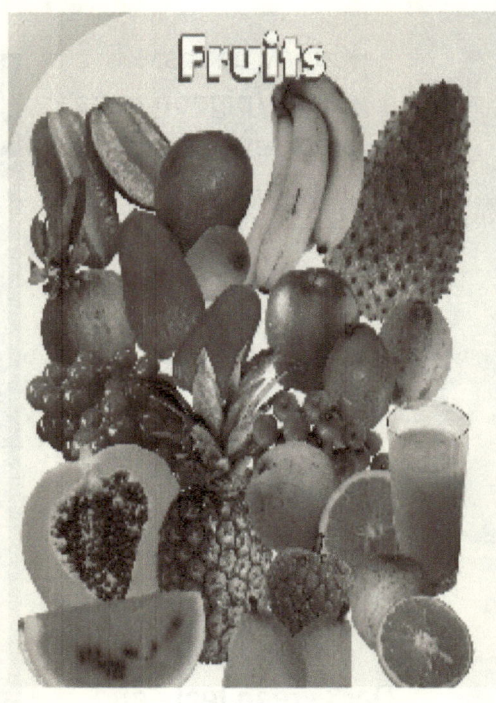

Mango, guava, citrus (orange, grapefruit, limes, tangerine), pineapple, West Indian cherry, pawpaw/papaya, golden apple/Jew/June plum, sugar apple/sweet sop.

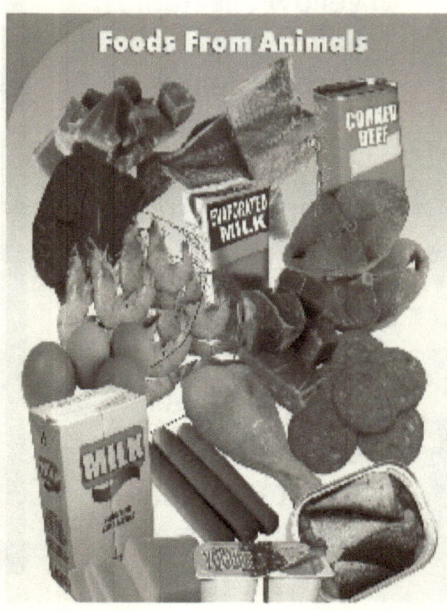

Meat, poultry, fish (fresh, canned, pickled, dried), milk, cheese, yoghurt, egg, liver, heart, kidney, tripe (offal), trotters, feet, tail, head

84

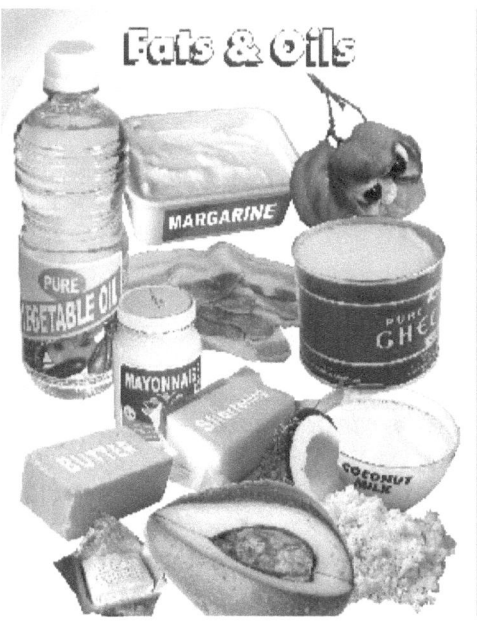

Fats & Oils

Cooking and salad oils, butter, margarine, shortening, ghee, coconut cream/milk, meat fat, nuts, avocado pear, Jamaican ackee.

Section C: Guide to Healthy Food Choices

Time allocated: 10 minutes

Teacher's activity:

- Distribute sample food labels to students
- Ask them to look out for the following areas as you explain to them. The areas are serving size, calories and nutrient facts panel.

Teaching aid: sample of food label Table 9.1.

Summary

These are some of the steps to follow for healthy food choices.

Check serving size

The serving size will show you exactly how many calories and nutrients you will be getting from the food (remember, a package may contain one or more than servings). Ask students to check serving sizes on sample labels and report.

<u>Consider the calories</u>

When looking at a food's calories: Remember! 100 = moderate, 400 = high NB: the food labels are based on a 2,000 calories diet, but individuals have different caloric needs.

<u>Choose nutrients wisely</u>

◈ Nutrients to get more of: potassium, fibre, vitamin A and C, iron and calcium

◈ *[Encourage students to choose foods with a higher %DV of these important nutrients.]*

◈ Nutrients to get less of: Trans fat, saturated fat, cholesterol, sodium and sugars. *[Remind students to choose foods that are lower in these nutrients']*

Teacher goes through the guide to healthy eating chart (below) with students.

Section D: Examine and Read Food Labels [Practical]

Time allocated: 10 minutes

Teaching aid: Ask students to take out favorite snack with labels to class.

Teaching activity: Guide students to examine and read the snack label

Summary

Based on the previous section (section C) guide students to read their food labels (see PowerPoint). The Nutrition Fact Panel is located on the outside of the package or box of food, such as the side of a cereal box, or the back of a package of macaroni. Work through the examples in the PowerPoint presentation.

Guide to Healthy Eating

FOOD GROUPS	POSITIVE CHOICES	NEGATIVE CHOICES
STAPLES	Ground provisions, whole wheat products, high fibre cereals, whole grain pastas	White flour products, pastries, deep fried root vegetables
LEGUMES	Fresh peas, dried peas and beans, unsalted nuts, baked nuts	Salted nuts, deep fried peas, beans, nuts, canned peas and beans, peas and beans cooked with salted butter, cured meats or margarine
DARK GREEN, LEAFY and YELLOW VEGETABLES	Fresh, steamed, grilled or baked vegetables	Vegetables in cream sauces, boiled or canned vegetables
FRUITS	Fresh fruit juices, fresh fruits, unsweetened juice	Fruits packed in syrup; juices made from concentrate, juice crystals

FOOD FROM ANIMALS	Skinless poultry, trimmed cuts of meat, seafood packed in spring water, egg whites, low fat or skimmed milk and dairy products, low fat cheeses	Sausages, egg yolks, red meats, fats of meats, canned or processed meats, skin of poultry, wing and foot of poultry, full cream milk, condensed milk, cheese spreads, lard, other animal fats, cured, smoked or salted meats and seafood, highly marbled meats, seafood packed in brine and artificial flavourings
FATS and OILS	Vegetable oils, soft spread margarines, low fat salad dressings, low fat/fat free mayonnaise dressings	Animal fats—bacon fat, lard, avocado, ghee, butter, regular salad dressings or mayonnaise dressings, regular sandwich spreads, cream, salted butter/ margarine

The key to using this guide for healthy eating is to remember that moderation is essential. Maintaining balance with regards to food intake, adequate water consumption, as well as physical activity levels are important considerations for healthy food and lifestyle choices.

Table 9.1. Sample Food Label

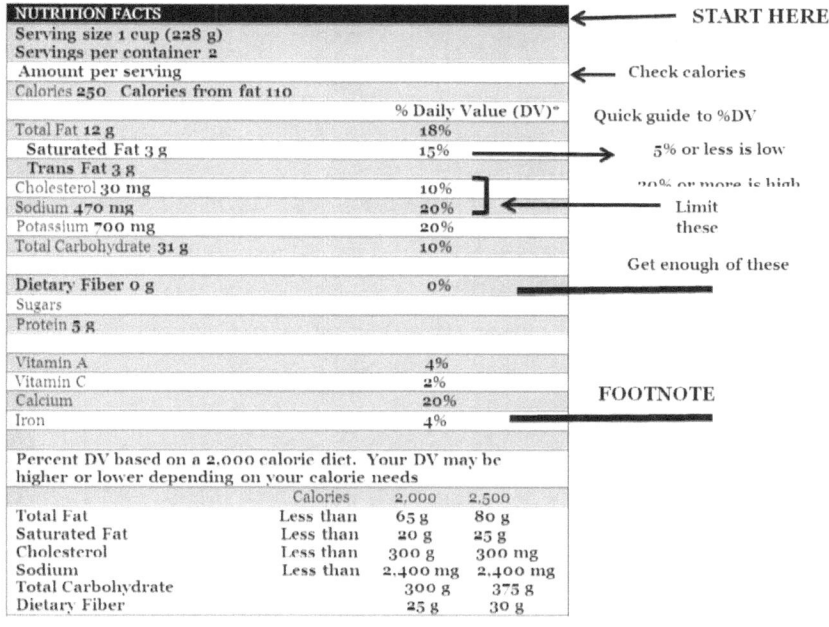

To read the label:

1. Start here ⟶ NUTRITION FACTS PANEL

NUTRITION FACTS
Serving size 1 cup (228 g)
Servings per container 2

❖ Start with the **NUTRITION FACTS** panel—most importantly:

❖ Know your serving size and number of servings in the package or can

❖ If the label says *"one cup"* per serving size and *"two servings per container"* that means there are two cups in the whole package or can

2. CHECK OUT THE TOTAL CALORIS AND FAT

Amount per serving
Calories **250** **Calories from fat 110**

❖ Calories provide a measure of how much energy you get from a serving of the food
❖ The calorie section of the label can help you manage your weight
❖ Remember, the number of servings you eat determines the number of calories you actually eat (your portion amount)

3. CHECK OUT THE TOTAL CALORIS AND FAT

Amount per serving
Calories **250** **Calories from fat 110**

Example: There are 250 calories in one serving of macaroni pie. How many calories from fat are there in ONE serving?

❖ The calorie section of the label can help you manage your weight
❖ Remember, the number of servings you eat determines the number of calories you actually eat (your portion amount)

Answer: 110 calories, which means almost half the calories in a single serving, come from fat. What if you ate the whole package content? Then you will consume two servings or 500 calories and 220 would come from fat.

4. THE NUTRIENTS—HOW MUCH?

❖ Look at the top of the nutrient section in the sample label

❖ It shows you some key nutrients that impact on your health and separates them into two main groups

Get Enough Vitamins, Minerals and Fibre		
Dietary Fiber 0 g	0%
Vitamin A	4%
Vitamin C	2%
Calcium	20%
Iron	4%

❖ Eat more dietary fibre, vitamins A and C, calcium and iron to maintain good health. Choose more fruits and vegetables to get more of these nutrients

❖ Remember, you can use the Nutrition Facts panel to increase those nutrients you want to consume enough of and limit those nutrients you want to cut back on

Limit Fat Cholesterol and Sodium		
Total Fat 12 g	18%
Saturated Fat 3 g	15%
Trans Fat 3 g	
Cholesterol 30 mg	10%
Sodium 470 mg	20%

❖ Eat less of these nutrients - fat, saturated fat, trans fat, cholesterol or sodium may help reduce your risk for certain chronic diseases like diabetes, heart disease, some types of cancer and high blood pressure.

5. Understanding the Footnote

Understanding the footnote on the bottom of the Nutrition Facts Panel

Percent DV based on a 2,000 calorie diet. Your DV may be higher or lower depending on your calorie needs			
	Calories	2,000	2,500
Total Fat	Less than	65 g	80 g
Saturated Fat	Less than	20 g	25 g
Cholesterol	Less than	300 g	300 mg
Sodium	Less than	2,400 mg	2,400 mg
Total Carbohydrate		300 g	375 g
Dietary Fiber		25 g	30 g

The footnote in the lower part of the nutrition label, which tells you "%DV are based on a 2,000 calorie diet" must be on all labels.

6. QUICK GUIDE TO %DV

% Daily Value (DV)*	
Total Fat 12 g	18%
Saturated Fat 3 g	15%
Trans Fat 3 g	
Cholesterol 30 mg	10%
Sodium 470 mg	20%
Potassium 700 mg	20%
Total Carbohydrate 31 g	10%
Dietary Fiber 0 g	0%
Sugars	
Protein 5 g	
Vitamin A	4%
Vitamin C	2%
Calcium	20%
Iron	4%

5 %DV is low and 20 %DV or more is high

This guide tells you that 5 %DV or less is low for all nutrients, those you want to limit (e.g. fat, cholesterol or sodium), or for those you want to consume in greater amounts (fibre etc.)

92

EVALUATION—DIABETES PREVENTION AND CONTROL—HEALTHY EATING

Name: _____   Maximum Points: 15

Instructions: Answer all Questions Correctly

Circle True or False for the sentences below

1. Calories are supplied by carbohydrates, proteins and fats.   . . . True   . . . False   *1 point*

2. . . . tells you if there is a lot or a little of a nutrient (like calcium) in a serving of food.   *1 point*

    a. Calories   b. % DVD   c. Serving size

3. Draw and label a healthy portion plate the Caribbean Food Groups.   *2 points*

4. Which food groups provide protein-rich foods?   *1 point*

    a. Food from animals, legumes
    b. Food from animals
    c. Legumes and vegetables
    d. Fruits and vegetables
    e. Fats and oils, food from animals
    f. Legumes and staples

5. Which food groups contain food that should be eaten in very small quantity?

    a. Food from animals
    b. Legumes
    c. Vegetables
    d. Staples
    e. Fats and oils   *1 point*

6. What is a balanced diet?   *1 point*
    a. Food eaten daily to provide most of the nutrients
    b. Eating foods that we like all the time
    c. Eating to correct any deficiency in our diet
    d. Contains all the food from the food group to meet our needs daily
    e. Everything we eat from our plate
7. Avocado falls in the category of   *1 point*
    a. Staples
    b. Legumes
    c. Vegetables
    d. Fats and oils
    e. Fruits
8. Staples provide mainly   *1 point*
    a. Carbohydrate
    b. Protein
    c. Fats
    d. Mineral
    e. Vitamin
9. **Instructions**: using the sample Nutritional Fact label on Nutrition Facts 1 and 2 (given).
    Fill out the blank spaces.   *3 points*
    a. <u>Nutrition Facts 1</u>   <u>Nutrition Facts 2</u>
       Calories . . . .   Calories . . . .
       Serving size . . . .   Serving size . . . .
       Total fat . . . .   Total fat . . . .
    b. Based on the nutritional fact, between the Facts 1 and the Facts 2, which one will you consume and why?   *3 points*

LESSON TEN

DIABETES PREVENTION AND
CONTROL—PHYSICAL ACTIVITY

Age level: 10-15 years   **Class time**: 45 minutes

Teaching Objectives

The objectives of this lesson are to:

◈ Create awareness of the benefits of physical activity for people at risk for diabetes, and for those with type I and type II diabetes

◈ Provide guidelines for healthy physical activity

Learning Outcomes

By the end of the lesson, students should be able to:

◈ List three benefits of physical activity for people with type 1 diabetes

◈ List three benefit of physical activity for people with type 2 diabetes

◈ Explain five guidelines for healthy physical activity

Relevant previous knowledge

◈ Overview of Nutrition

◈ Carbohydrate Digestion

◈ Overview of Diabetes

◈ Complications in Diabetes

◈ Diabetes Prevention and Control—Healthy Eating

Introduction

Time allocated: 5 minutes

Teaching method: Lecture

Teaching activity: teacher reviews previous lessons and introduces the final lesson.

Summary

In the final lesson of this primer, we will talk about the importance of physical activity in diabetes prevention and management. So far, in our diabetes prevention and management lessons, we have looked at nutrition and nutrients with emphases on carbohydrate and its digestion; we have also studied about diabetes; complications in diabetes; and healthy eating.

Section A—Definition of Physical Activity

Time: 5 minutes

Teaching method: Class discussion

Teaching activity: Teacher ask the students *what they know about physical activity and have them list some examples of physical activity they do.*

Summary

Physical activity is usually done to develop or maintain physical fitness and overall health. Being physically active is essential for the good health of everyone and may reduce your risk of Type 2 diabetes. Also, it is especially helpful for people with diabetes. It improves the way their body feels and reduces stress.

What counts as activity?

Every form of physical activity counts (for example, walking, jogging, aerobic dancing, bicycling, swimming etc.). The recommended minimum amount of activity for:

- ◆ Adults—30 minutes on at least five days of the week (that is only 2.5 hours out of a 168 hour week)
- ◆ Children—one hour per day

Activity can be spread out through the day into bite-size chunks. We are all recommended to achieve at least 10,000 steps a day. Why not consider buying a pedometer to log how many steps you take?

Section B—Benefits of Physical Activity for Type 1 Diabetes

Time allocated: 6 minutes

Teaching method: Discussion

Teaching activity: Teacher asks students: *How do you feel after being physically active?*

Summary

Why is keeping active important to you?

Many people enjoy being active not just for their health, but because it makes them feel better and helps stop their weight creeping up. You may want to ask yourself what being more active means to you. Some people say it makes them more mobile, less out of breath, less stressed and helps them sleep better. Well, there are a number of health benefits to keeping physically active. It will:

- ◈ Reduce the risk of Type 2 diabetes, stroke or heart attack
- ◈ Help lower blood pressure
- ◈ Improve your cholesterol levels
- ◈ Strengthen your bones

Benefits of exercise for people with Type 1 diabetes

- ◈ It improves the action of insulin in the body
- ◈ It reduces fats in the blood
- ◈ It lowers high blood pressure

- Being active helps the body to use insulin more efficiently, and regular activity can help reduce the amount of insulin your child takes.
- Being active helps your child maintain a healthy weight for their height, which in turn will assist their diabetes control

Section C—Benefits of Exercise for Type 2 Diabetes

Time Allocated: 6 minutes

Teaching method: Discussion

Summary

Benefit of exercise for people with type II diabetes

- Physical activity increases the amount of glucose used by the muscles for energy, so it may sometimes lower blood glucose levels.
- It reduces fats in the blood
- It lowers high blood pressure
- It decrease fat in the body
- It builds muscle tissue

Note: exercise can lower the blood glucose for 16 to 24 hours after the actual exercise. Even a little exercise can make a big difference in diabetes control.

Section D—Guidelines for Exercise and Diabetes

Time allocate: 6 minutes

Teaching method: Lecture

Summary

1. Build up gradually. If you have been inactive for a number of years your body may take time to adjust as your heart and muscles tone up.

2. Set yourself daily, weekly and monthly goals or targets.
3. Try keeping a physical activity journal to monitor your progress and reward yourself for achieving your goals.
4. Try varying your activity to avoid boredom setting in, and do not be afraid to try new activities.
5. Do not give up. Although your body benefits as soon as you become more active you may not see visible changes straight away. After a few weeks the benefits will become more noticeable to you.
6. Regular habits included in your daily routine are easier to achieve.
7. If you find an activity you enjoy, you are more likely to keep it up. Better still, try taking up an activity the whole family or your friends can enjoy.
• Drink plenty of water before and after exercise to avoid becoming thirsty.

Evaluation (see next page)

Time allocated: 10 minutes

Closure

Time allocated: 7 minutes

Teaching activity: teacher summarizes the lesson and invites questions from students.

EVALUATION—DIABETES PREVENTION AND CONTROL—PHYSICAL ACTIVITY

Name: _____   Maximum Points: 10

Instructions: Answer all Questions Correctly

Circle True or False for the sentences below

1. Physical activity is done to develop
   or maintain physical fitness and
   overall health.   . . . True   . . . False   *1 point*

2. List three benefit of physical activity for people with type I diabetes
   a. _____
   b. _____
   c. _____ *3 points*

3. List three benefit of physical activity for people with type II diabetes
   a. _____
   b. _____
   c. _____ *3 points*

4. List three guidelines to effective physical activity
   a. _____
   b. _____
   c. _____ *3 points*

LESSON ELEVEN—OVERALL EVALUATION

Evaluation Questions to choose from
SET I—20 Points
1. Nutrition is the study of foods and nutrients are the
   _____ in food.   *2 points*
       a. Components b. Compromises c. Confidences
2. List the six classes of nutrients   *6 points*
       a. C_____   W_____
       b. P_____   V_____
       c. F_____   M_____
3. Food performs all the following functions
   EXCEPT: *2 points*
       a. Growth
       b. Repair
       c. Energize
       d. Operate
       e. Protect
4. **Circle True or False for the sentence below**:
       a. A balanced diet should be
           in the right proportion
           and amount   . . . True   . . . False *2 points*
5. List three risk factors for chronic disease
   development   *6 points*
       a. _____
       b. _____
       c. _____

6. Diabetes is as disease that affects the
body's use of   *2 points*
    a. Water   b. Glucose   c. Vitamins

SET II—25 POINTS

Circle True or False for the sentences below

1. Carbohydrate provides the
body with energy.   . . . True   . . . False *2 points*

2. Carbohydrates can be simple
or complex.   . . . True   . . . False *2 points*

3. Simple carbohydrates are quickly broken
down to glucose.   . . . True   . . . False *2 points*

4. Digestion allows our bodies to get the nutrients
and energy it needs from the
food we eat.   . . . True   . . . False *1 point*

Fill in the blanks

5. Complex carbohydrates include
                    . . . . and . . . .   *1 point*

6. Dietary fiber can be classified as
                    . . . . and . . . .   *1 point*

7. Using the food list and table below, classify the
given foods as complex or simple carbohydrates.
Food list: sweets, cakes, syrup, bubble gum, soft
drink, oatmeal, sweet potatoes, dried peas and
beans, Kit Kat, wheat bread, white bread, ice cream
and sweet biscuits, macaroni, corn   *15 points*

SIMPLE CARBOHYDRATES	COMPLEX CARBOHYDRATES

SET III—25 Points
Circle True or False for the sentences below

1. There are animal and plant sources
   of protein.   . . . True   . . . False   *1 point*

2. Protein is essential to
   good health.   . . . True   . . . False   *1 point*

3. Protein always means
   red meat.   . . . True   . . . False   *1 point*

4. Fats in our foods that come
   from plants are liquid at
   room temperature.   . . . True   . . . False   *1 point*

5. Vegetable shortenings, which are plant
   oils remain solid at
   room temperature.   . . . True   . . . False   *1 point*

6. A liquid is something that can flow
   and take on the shape
   of its container.   . . . True   . . . False   *1 point*

7. List three reasons why protein is
   needed by the body.   *3 points*

   _____

   _____

   _____

   _____

8. Complete the chart by listing as many foods containing protein as you can. Identify the sources of protein as either animal or plant. *6 points*

Food containing Protein	Source

9. List three reasons why we need lipids in the body *6 points*

   a. _____

   b. _____

   c. _____

10. What are lipids? *4 points*

SET IV—25 Points

1. Name the functions of at least five vitamins *10 points*

2. List at least two food sources of five vitamins *10 points*

Fill in the blanks

3. Vitamins _____ are water-soluble. *3 points*

4. The fat soluble vitamins are

   _____ *2 points*

SET V—25 Points

1. There are about _____ different minerals that make up about _____ of our bodies. *3 points*

2. Minerals are also divided into two groups.
   They are: *4 points*
   a.
   b.
3. The macro-minerals are
   _____   *2 points*
4. The trace-minerals are
   _____   *2 points*
5. Using the table below, fill in the functions
   and food sources of each mineral named
   in the first column   *14 points*

MINERAL	FUNCTION	SOURCES
Calcium		
Phosphorus		
Potassium		
Sodium		
Iron		

Zinc		
Iodine		
Fibre Roughage Cellulose		

SET VI—25 Points

Circle True or False for the sentences below.

1. Digestion allows our bodies to get the nutrients and energy it needs from the food we eat. . . . True . . . False *4 points*

2. Glucose is the main fuel for the body. . . . True . . . False *3 points*

Fill in the blanks using the given words

3. Carbohydrate digestions begin in the . . . .

   a. Nose   b. stomach   c. mouth   *4 points*

4. Glucose is the end product of . . . .

   a. Carbohydrates   b. fat   c. protein   *4 points*

Match the following pairs correctly:

a.	Mouth	Insulin
b.	Liver	Salivary gland
c.	Pancreas	Gall bladder
d.	Small intestines	Excretion
e.	Rectum	Absorption *10 points*

SET VII—25 Points

Circle True or False for the sentences below.

1. Glucose comes from digestion
   of carbohydrates. . . . True . . . False *1 point*

2. Type I diabetes usually occurs
   in children. . . . True . . . False *1 point*

3. Type II diabetes is caused by
   eating sweets. . . . True . . . False *1 point*

4. All overweight people will
   get diabetes. . . . True . . . False *1 point*

5. Diabetes is a disease that involves
   blood sugar levels. . . . True . . . False *1 point*

6. Healthy eating is one treatment for
   type 2 diabetes. . . . True . . . False *1 point*

Fill in the blanks

7. Diabetes is a disease that affects the
   body's use of . . . . *2 points*
   a. Water   b. Glucose   c. Vitamins

8. Glucose is used by the body and
   turned into . . . . *2 points*
   a. Energy   b. Starch   c. Carbohydrates

9. The pancreas makes a
   hormone called . . . . *2 points*
   a. Growth hormone b. Insulin c. Thyroid hormone

10. Lemons are to oranges as
    sugar is to . . . . *2 points*
    a. Hormones   b. Salt   c. Glucose   d. Juice

11. List 5 symptoms of diabetes. *11 points*

_____

_____

_____

_____

_____

SET VIII—25 Points

Circle True or False for the sentences below.

1. Hypoglycemia is high
   blood sugar.   . . . True   . . . False *1 point*
2. Hyperglycemia is high
   blood sugar.   . . . True   . . . False *1 point*

Instructions: Check the correct answer(s) *15 points*

3. Hypoglycemia can be caused by:
   a. . . . Eating too little food
   b. . . . Talking to a friend
   c. . . . Delaying a meal
   d. . . . Doing more exercise than you normally do
4. Hyperglycemia can be caused by:
   a. . . . Eating foods containing too much
      carbohydrates
   b. . . . Infections
   c. . . . Talking in class
   d. . . . Not producing enough insulin
5. The following are symptoms of
   hypoglycemia **EXCEPT**   *4 points*
      a. Anger b. Sweating c. Shakiness d. Salivating

6. The following are symptoms of
   hyperglycemia **EXCEPT**
   a. Inability to speak. b. Drowsiness c. Dry mouth
   d. Dry throat   *4 points*

SET IX—25 Points
Circle True or False for the sentences below
1. Calories are supplied by carbohydrates,
   proteins and fats.   . . . True   . . . False *1 point*
2. . . . tells you if there is a lot or a little of a nutrient
   (like calcium) in a serving of food.   *1 point*
   a. Calories   b. % DVD   c. Serving size
3. Draw and label a healthy plate of the
   Caribbean Food Groups.   *2 points*
4. What areas do you look out for on the
   nutrition fact label on food in order to make
   wise healthy choices?   *1 point*
   a. Serving size b. Calories c. Nutrients d   .
   Weight
5. Which food groups provide
   protein-rich foods?   *1 point*
   a. Food from animals, legumes
   b. Food from animals
   c. Legumes and vegetables
   d. Fruits and vegetables
   e. Fats and oils, food from animals
   f. Legumes and staples

6. Which food groups contain food that should be eaten in very small quantity?
    a. Food from animals
    b. Legumes
    c. Vegetables
    d. Staples
    e. Fats and oils   *1 point*
7. What is a balanced diet?   *1 point*
    a. Food eaten daily to provide most of the nutrients
    b. Eating foods that we like all the time
    c. Eating to correct any deficiency in our diet
    d. Contains all the food from the food group to meet our needs daily
    e. Everything we eat from our plate
8. Avocado falls in the category of   *1 point*
    a. a. Staple
    b. Legumes
    c. Vegetables
    d. Fats and oils
    e. Fruits
9. Staples provide mainly provide   *1 point*
    a. Carbohydrate
    b. Protein
    c. Fats
    d. Mineral
    e. Vitamin

Instructions: using the sample Nutritional Fact label on Nutrition Facts 1 and 2 (given). Fill out the blank spaces. *10 points*

10. Nutrition Facts 1   Nutrition Facts 2

    a. Calories . . . .   Calories . . . .

    b. Serving size . . . .   Serving size . . . .

    c. Total fat . . . .   Total fat . . . .

11. Based on the nutritional fact, between the Facts 1 and the Facts 2, which one will you consume and why? *6 points*

Vitamin Study Sheet

Name: _____

1. Vitamins are found in: _____.

2. Vitamins do not provide _____,
   but they are essential because
   they _____.

3. Vitamins cannot be _____
   by our bodies. They must be _____
   or _____ in our food.

4. Vitamins assist the body in using food by _____
   _____

5. Vitamins are divided into two groups:
   a.
   b.

6. Examples of the two groups of vitamins are:
   a.
   b.

7. Fat-soluble vitamins are transported through the
   body by what method?
   _____

8. Water-soluble are transported through the body by
   what method?
   _____

9. Name the main function of Vitamin C.
   _____

10. Name two main sources for Vitamin D. _____
    and _____.

11. Match the following vitamins with their function.

_____ 1. Vitamin C   A. Strong bones . . . from the sun

_____ 2. Vitamin A   B. For good vision

_____ 3. Vitamin D   C. Prevents scurvy

VITAMIN STUDY SHEET

Vitamin and Mineral Bingo

Available at http://www.uen.org; accessed 9/29/2013

Name: _____

Teacher's activity: Teacher fits in vitamins and minerals words and have students play bingo

			FREE	
		FREE		
	FREE			

Vitamin and Mineral Bingo

Name: _____

			FREE	
		FREE		
	FREE			

My Favorite Physical Activities

Name: _____

Make a list of your favorite Outdoor Activities
Now, circle the activities that will help your heart and bones
stay strong:
Fishing
Hiking
Tennis
Running
Walking
Video games
Jogging
Homework
Cricket
Jump rope
Television
Text messaging
Listening to music
Football
Dance

FOOD LABEL REFERENCE GUIDE

Name: _____

Watch out for servings per container, calories, fat, trans fat, cholesterol and sodium

Look for foods high in fibre, vitamin A, Vitamin C, calcium and iron

NUTRITION FACTS	
Serving size 1 cup (228 g)	
Servings per container 2	
Amount per serving	
Calories 250 Calories from fat 110	
% Daily Value (DV)*	
Total Fat 12 g	18%
Saturated Fat 3 g	15%
Trans Fat 3 g	
Cholesterol 30 mg	10%
Sodium 470 mg	20%
Potassium 700 mg	20%
Total Carbohydrate 31 g	10%
Dietary Fiber 0 g	0%
Sugars	
Protein 5 g	
Vitamin A	4%
Vitamin C	2%
Calcium	20%
Iron	4%

Percent DV based on a 2,000 calorie diet. Your DV may be higher or lower depending on your calorie needs

Use the 5% and 20% rule

5% is low and 20% is high for any of these nutrients.

NUTRITION FACTS LABEL ACTIVITY

COMPARE FOOD LABELS WORKSHEET

Teacher's activity: Have the students cut-out and bring to school food labels from packaged food items. Have the students trade food labels with their classmates so that each student has two food labels. Have the student use their food labels to fill out the Food Label Worksheet. *Write in the name of the Food Labels you are using. Name of Food Label A Name of Food Label B*

	Write the name of the food label you are using
Name of Food Label A	
Name of Food Label B	

Circle your food label that is best described

1.	Most sodium per serving	Label A	Label B
2.	Most carbohydrate per serving	Label A	Label B
3.	Most saturated fat per serving	Label A	Label B
4.	Most sugar per serving	Label A	Label B
5.	Most calories per serving	Label A	Label B
6.	Most fat per serving	Label A	Label B
7.	Has less sodium	Label A	Label B

8. Least amount of calories per serving	Label A	Label B
9. Most protein per serving	Label A	Label B
10. Most total fat per serving	Label A	Label B
11. Most vitamin A	Label A	Label B
12. Most calcium	Label A	Label B

Which food item do you think is more healthy and why?

_____

_____

_____

_____

_____

_____

_____

_____

_____

Diabetes Concentration Game

(Available at https://www.education.mihs.org/diabetes; accessed 9/29/2013)

Name: _____

Objective: Given a set of diabetes related picture and word cards, the students will be able to identify and distinguish the different terms associated with diabetes.

Materials: 2 copies of Diabetes Concentration cards per group of 2 students (heavy tag board works best).

Activity: 1) Give each group of two students 2 copies of Diabetes Concentration and have them carefully cut them out; 2) Have the students shuffle their cards and lay them picture side down on the floor or table 3) The students take turns flipping over one card, followed by one more in hopes of matching the first card. Each time they flip a card over they must say the name on the card. If the second card does not match the first they must turn the cards face down and it is then the next person's turn. If the student gets a matching pair they keep that pair and may repeat their turn until they do not have a matching pair. 4) Play until all the cards have been matched. Students with the most matched pairs wins!

Evaluation: After playing several times, have students construct eight complete sentences correctly using the diabetes-related definitions. Class may share answers upon completion.

These cards will be on the left hand side of the playing surface face down.

DIABETES	GLUCOSE	PANCREAS
INSULIN	HORMONE	BLOODSTREAM
SYMPTOMS	GENETIC	HEALTHY WEIGHT
INACTIVITY INJECTIONS	COMPLICATIONS RESPONSIBILITY	EXERCISE FRUITS AND VEGETABLES
GRAINS	DAIRY	Caribbean Six Food Groups
CALORIES	HEALTHY BEVERAGES	REGULAR CHECKUPS

These cards will be on the right hand side of the playing surface face down.

A disease that affects how the body uses glucose	A sugar our body uses for energy	Organ that makes the hormone *insulin*
Hormone produced by the pancreas	Substance created by the body's organs	Carries needed minerals and nutrients throughout the body
An indication of a disease or other disorder	Occurring among members of a family	A persons normal weight according to their height and age
Passive or not moving	Negative things that can occur from diabetes	Bodily training for the improvement of health
Introduced into the body by a syringe	Having reliability or dependability	Mango, oranges, cabbage, carrots

Good source of fiber	Milk, yoghurt, cheese	Food groups of a healthy diet
The energy value of food	Water, low fat milk, no sweet drink	Visit your doctor often

RESOURCES USED

- KidsHealth.org/classroom
- Food and Health Communication www.Foodand Health.com
- www.fda.gov/spottheblock
- Changing Diabetes-us.com
- American Diabetes Association: http://www.diabetes. org/living-withdiabetes/treatment-and-care/ blood-glucose-control.html
- Exercise and diabetes, medical information from "the Cleveland Clinic", edited by Charlotte E. Grayson. MD, Nov.2002. "WebMDHealth."
- Diabetes Association of Trinidad and Tobago (DATT)
- Diabetes UK
- PAHO (Pan American Health Organization). (2006). Managing diabetes in primary care in the Caribbean. Office of Caribbean Programme Coordination, PAHO, Barbados.
- THSI (Trinidad and Tobago Health Sciences Initiative). (2009). Centre of Excellence for Diabetes Services and Training. http://www.tthsi.org.tt/index. php?page_key=73&column2=1 (accessed 01/19/12)
- Ministry of Health 2011 National Risk factor Survey—STEPS-http://www.health.gov.tt (accessed 01/19/12)

- Lorig, K., González, VM. (2000). Community-based diabetes self-management education: Definition and case study. Diabetes Spectrum 13, 234.
- Jacobs, J. 2011. Has the USDA written a standardized definition for a serving size? http://www.livestrong.com/article/529913-has-the-usda-written-a-standardized-definition-for-a-serving-size/#ixzz26iSVE9rv
- Brown, S. The Caribbean food groups. Available at http://zunal.com/webquest.php?w=67056; accessed September 17th, 2012.
- *http://www.cdc.gov/healthyweight/assessing/bmi/childrens_bmi/about_childrens_bmi.html*
- The glucose molecule. Available at: getfitnesstogether.wordpress.com (Accessed October 2, 2012).
- Organic, Biochemistry, Chapter 25. In: Chemistry in perspective. Adrian Faiers MA (Oxon) MCIPR. Available at: http://www.csb.yale.edu/userguides/graphics/msp/cpk.html; accessed October 2nd, 2012.
- Pereira, LMP, Da Silva, CK, Teelucksingh, S. 2009. Are current guidelines addressing the diabetes challenge in the Caribbean? Asia-Pacific J Endocrinology 1: (1), October.

www.ingramcontent.com/pod-product-compliance
Lightning Source LLC
Chambersburg PA
CBHW022010170526
45157CB00003B/1217